BIOMEDICAL DEVICES AND THEIR APPLICATIONS

AF849084

MEDICAL DEVICES AND THE FDA

REGULATION, USER FEES AND TORT CLAIMS

BIOMEDICAL DEVICES AND THEIR APPLICATIONS

Additional books in this series can be found on Nova's website under the Series tab.

Additional E-books in this series can be found on Nova's website under the E-book tab.

LAWS AND LEGISLATION

Additional books in this series can be found on Nova's website under the Series tab.

Additional E-books in this series can be found on Nova's website under the E-book tab.

BIOMEDICAL DEVICES AND THEIR APPLICATIONS

MEDICAL DEVICES AND THE FDA

REGULATION, USER FEES AND TORT CLAIMS

GIL FRAZIER
AND
BRADY MALONE
EDITORS

nova
publishers
New York

Copyright © 2013 by Nova Science Publishers, Inc.

All rights reserved. No part of this book may be reproduced, stored in a retrieval system or transmitted in any form or by any means: electronic, electrostatic, magnetic, tape, mechanical photocopying, recording or otherwise without the written permission of the Publisher.

For permission to use material from this book please contact us:
Telephone 631-231-7269; Fax 631-231-8175
Web Site: http://www.novapublishers.com

NOTICE TO THE READER

The Publisher has taken reasonable care in the preparation of this book, but makes no expressed or implied warranty of any kind and assumes no responsibility for any errors or omissions. No liability is assumed for incidental or consequential damages in connection with or arising out of information contained in this book. The Publisher shall not be liable for any special, consequential, or exemplary damages resulting, in whole or in part, from the readers' use of, or reliance upon, this material. Any parts of this book based on government reports are so indicated and copyright is claimed for those parts to the extent applicable to compilations of such works.

Independent verification should be sought for any data, advice or recommendations contained in this book. In addition, no responsibility is assumed by the publisher for any injury and/or damage to persons or property arising from any methods, products, instructions, ideas or otherwise contained in this publication.

This publication is designed to provide accurate and authoritative information with regard to the subject matter covered herein. It is sold with the clear understanding that the Publisher is not engaged in rendering legal or any other professional services. If legal or any other expert assistance is required, the services of a competent person should be sought. FROM A DECLARATION OF PARTICIPANTS JOINTLY ADOPTED BY A COMMITTEE OF THE AMERICAN BAR ASSOCIATION AND A COMMITTEE OF PUBLISHERS.

Additional color graphics may be available in the e-book version of this book.

Library of Congress Cataloging-in-Publication Data

ISBN: 978-1-62257-674-6

Published by Nova Science Publishers, Inc. † New York

CONTENTS

PREFACE

Medical device regulation is complex, in part because of the wide variety of items that are categorized as medical devices. They may be simple tools used during medical examinations, such as tongue depressors and thermometers, or high-tech life-saving implants like heart valves and coronary stents. The medical device market has been characterized as including eight industry sectors: surgical and medical instrument manufacturing, surgical appliance and supplies, in vitro diagnostic products (IVDs, or laboratory tests), electromedical and electrotherapeutic apparatus, irradiation apparatus, dental equipment and supplies, ophthalmic goods, and dental laboratories. This book explores FDA regulation of medical devices with a focus on the user fee program and tort claims.

Chapter 1 - Prior to and since the passage of the Medical Device Amendments of 1976, Congress has debated how best to ensure that consumers have access, as quickly as possible, to new and improved medical devices and, at the same time, prevent devices that are not safe and effective from entering or remaining on the market. Medical devices regulation is complex, in part, because of the wide variety of items that are categorized as medical devices; examples range from a simple tongue depressor to a life-sustaining heart valve. The regulation of medical devices can affect their cost, quality, and availability in the health care system.

In order to be legally marketed in the United States, many medical devices must be reviewed by the Food and Drug Administration (FDA), the agency responsible for protecting the public health by overseeing medical products, including devices. FDA's Center for Devices and Radiological Health (CDRH) is primarily responsible for medical device review. CDRH activities are funded through a combination of public money (i.e., direct FDA appropriations from Congress) and private money (i.e., user fees collected from device manufacturers) which together comprise FDA's total. User fees account for 33% of FDA's total FY2011 program level and 15% of CDRH's program level, which is $378 million in FY2011 including $56 million in user fees. FDA's authority to collect user fees, originally authorized in 2002 (P.L. 107-250), has been reauthorized in five-year increments. It will expire on October 1, 2012, under the terms of the Medical Device User Fee Act of 2007 (MDUFA), Title II of the FDA Amendments Act of 2007 (FDAAA, P.L. 110-85).

FDA requires all medical product manufacturers to register their facilities, list their devices with FDA, and follow general controls requirements. FDA classifies devices according to the risk they pose to consumers. Premarket review is required for moderate- and high-risk devices. There are two paths that manufacturers can use to bring such devices to market. One path consists of conducting clinical studies, submitting a *premarket approval* (PMA) application and requires evidence providing reasonable assurance that the device is safe and effective. The other path involves submitting a *510(k) notification* demonstrating that the device is *substantially equivalent* to a device already on the market (*a predicate device*) that does not require a PMA. The 510(k) process results in FDA clearance and tends to be much less expensive and less time-consuming than seeking FDA approval via PMA. Substantial equivalence is determined by comparing the performance characteristics of a new device with those of a predicate device; clinical data demonstrating safety and effectiveness are usually not required. Once approved or cleared for marketing, manufacturers must comply with regulations on manufacturing, labeling, surveillance, device tracking, and adverse event reporting.

Problems related to medical devices can have serious consequences for consumers. Defects in medical devices, such as artificial hips and pacemakers, have caused severe patient injuries and deaths. In 2006, FDA reported 116,086 device-related injuries, 96,485 malfunctions, and 2,830 deaths; an analysis by the National Research Center for Women & Families claims there were 4,556 device-related deaths in 2009. Reports published in 2009 through 2011—by the Government Accountability Office (GAO), the Department of Health and Human Services Office of the Inspector General and the Institute of Medicine—have voiced concerns about FDA's device review process. In 2009 and 2011 GAO included FDA's oversight of medical products on the GAO list of high-risk areas. FDA has conducted internal reviews as well and is implementing changes.

Chapter 2 - The Food and Drug Administration (FDA) is the agency responsible for the regulation of medical devices. These are a wide range of products that are used to diagnose, treat, monitor, or prevent a disease or condition in a patient. A company must obtain FDA's prior approval or clearance before marketing many medical devices in the United States. The Center for Devices and Radiological Health (CDRH) within FDA is primarily responsible for medical device review and regulation.

Congress first gave FDA the authority to collect user fees from medical device companies in the Medical Device User Fee and Modernization Act of 2002 (P.L. 107-250). The purpose of the user fee program is to help reduce the time in which FDA can review and make decisions on marketing applications. Lengthy review times affect the industry, which waits to market its products, and patients, who wait to use these products. The user fee law provides a revenue stream for FDA; in conjunction, the agency negotiates with industry to set *performance goals* for the premarket review of medical devices. Reauthorization of FDA's medical device user fees last occurred in 2007, just before the FDA's authority would expire, via the Medical Device User Fee Amendments of 2007 (MDUFA II). Current authority will expire on October 1, 2012.

On February 1, 2012, FDA announced that it had reached "an agreement in principle" with the medical device industry on proposed recommendations for the second reauthorization—referred to as MDUFA III. A draft MDUFA III package, composed of statutory language and the FDA-industry agreement on performance goals and procedures, was posted on the FDA website on March 14, 2012, and a public meeting describing the draft was held on March 28, 2012. The 30-day comment period on the draft ended April 16, 2012. Following review of the comments, FDA may revise the recommendation and then is to submit the final package to Congress.

Since medical device user fees were first collected in FY2003, they have comprised an increasing proportion of FDA's device budget. Medical device user fees have raised a number of concerns, prompting Congress to carefully consider issues such as which agency activities could use fees, how user fees can be kept from supplanting federal funding, and which companies should qualify as a small business and pay a reduced fee.

Congress is also considering reauthorization of the Prescription Drug User Fee Act (PDUFA) as well as new proposals for a Generic Drug User Fee Act and a Biosimilars User Fee Act. It is likely that these three will be combined with MDUFA III along with a variety of related and unrelated issues. Because of the importance of user fees to FDA's budget, PDUFA and MDUFA are considered to be "must pass" legislation, and Congress has often in the past included language to address a range of other concerns. For example, MDUFA II included provisions about the extent to which FDA can delegate activities to third parties, a unique device identification system, and reporting requirements for devices linked to serious injuries or deaths. House and Senate committees are circulating discussion drafts that contain many proposals that would affect medical device regulation. FDA has indicated that some of these pending reforms could conflict with what was negotiated with industry in the MDUFA III proposal. Some reforms are of concern because they would require more agency resources; others were discussed during the user fee negotiations and were set aside. If MDUFA reauthorization does not occur by early summer, federal regulations require that reduction-in-force notices be sent out in July 2012, giving 60 days' advance notice to about 250 FDA employees that their employment under the MDUFA program would end September 30, 2012.

Chapter 3 - In *Riegel v. Medtronic, Inc.*, the United States Supreme Court held in an 8 to 1 decision that if the Food and Drug Administration (FDA) grants premarket approval (PMA) to a medical device, the device manufacturer is immune from certain suits under state tort law, due to an express preemption provision in the Medical Device Amendments of 1976 (MDA). This holding establishes that FDA PMA preempts claims such as strict liability, breach of implied warranty, and negligence in design, testing, manufacturing, labeling, distribution, sale, inspection, or marketing of the device to the extent that such state law claims are "different from, or in addition to" federal PMA requirements. However, the Supreme Court held that the MDA's express preemption provision did not prohibit state "claims premised on a violation of FDA regulation." The Court stated that such claims "'parallel,' rather than add to, federal requirements." Post-*Riegel*, the lower courts have come to differing conclusions when determining whether particular state law claims, such as manufacturing defect claims, "parallel" federal requirements, and thus are not preempted, or rather are state requirements "different from, or in addition to" federal requirements, and thus are preempted under *Riegel*.

The Supreme Court's decision has been a cause for concern for some Members of Congress who disagree with the ruling, as well as trial lawyers and patients. However, advocates of more limited tort liability, including the previous Administration, agree with the ruling. The decision has broad implications for consumers of Class III medical devices, who are prevented from suing device manufacturers on most state common law claims, as well as manufacturers, who are shielded from many suits if their device receives FDA

PMA. In the 111th Congress, bills were introduced—H.R. 1346, H.R. 4816, and S. 540—that would have overturned the Court's decision in *Riegel* by modifying the statute at issue. As of the date of this report, similar legislation has not been introduced in the 112th Congress.

This report will provide a brief overview of federal premarket regulation of medical devices. The report then provides an overview of federal preemption of state law, as well as arguments for and against federal preemption of state law tort claims with respect to medical devices. The report explains the Supreme Court's decision in *Riegel* and examines the concurring and dissenting opinions. Finally, the report analyzes the legal, procedural, policy, and legislative implications for Congress, consumers, and medical device manufacturers.

In: Medical Devices and the FDA ISBN: 978-1-62257-674-6
Editors: Gil Frazier and Brady Malone © 2013 Nova Science Publishers, Inc.

Chapter 1

FDA REGULATION OF MEDICAL DEVICES*

Judith A. Johnson

On June 20, 2012, the House of Representatives passed, by voice vote and under suspension of the rules, S. 3187 (EAH), the Food and Drug Administration Safety and Innovation Act, as amended. This bill would reauthorize the FDA prescription drug and medical device user fee programs (which would otherwise expire on September 30, 2012), create new user fee programs for generic and biosimilar drug approvals, and make other revisions to other FDA drug and device approval processes. It reflects bicameral compromise on earlier versions of the bill (S. 3187 [ES], which passed the Senate on May 24, 2012, and H.R. 5651 [EH], which passed the House on May 30, 2012).

SUMMARY

Prior to and since the passage of the Medical Device Amendments of 1976, Congress has debated how best to ensure that consumers have access, as quickly as possible, to new and improved medical devices and, at the same time, prevent devices that are not safe and effective from entering or remaining on the market. Medical devices regulation is complex, in part,

* This is an edited, reformatted and augmented version of the Congressional Research Service Publication, CRS Report for Congress R42130, dated June 25, 2012.

because of the wide variety of items that are categorized as medical devices; examples range from a simple tongue depressor to a life-sustaining heart valve. The regulation of medical devices can affect their cost, quality, and availability in the health care system.

In order to be legally marketed in the United States, many medical devices must be reviewed by the Food and Drug Administration (FDA), the agency responsible for protecting the public health by overseeing medical products, including devices. FDA's Center for Devices and Radiological Health (CDRH) is primarily responsible for medical device review. CDRH activities are funded through a combination of public money (i.e., direct FDA appropriations from Congress) and private money (i.e., user fees collected from device manufacturers) which together comprise FDA's total. User fees account for 33% of FDA's total FY2011 program level and 15% of CDRH's program level, which is $378 million in FY2011 including $56 million in user fees. FDA's authority to collect user fees, originally authorized in 2002 (P.L. 107-250), has been reauthorized in five-year increments. It will expire on October 1, 2012, under the terms of the Medical Device User Fee Act of 2007 (MDUFA), Title II of the FDA Amendments Act of 2007 (FDAAA, P.L. 110-85).

FDA requires all medical product manufacturers to register their facilities, list their devices with FDA, and follow general controls requirements. FDA classifies devices according to the risk they pose to consumers. Premarket review is required for moderate- and high-risk devices. There are two paths that manufacturers can use to bring such devices to market. One path consists of conducting clinical studies, submitting a *premarket approval* (PMA) application and requires evidence providing reasonable assurance that the device is safe and effective. The other path involves submitting a *510(k) notification* demonstrating that the device is *substantially equivalent* to a device already on the market (*a predicate device*) that does not require a PMA. The 510(k) process results in FDA clearance and tends to be much less expensive and less time-consuming than seeking FDA approval via PMA. Substantial equivalence is determined by comparing the performance characteristics of a new device with those of a predicate device; clinical data demonstrating safety and effectiveness are usually not required. Once approved or cleared for marketing, manufacturers must comply with regulations on manufacturing, labeling, surveillance, device tracking, and adverse event reporting.

Problems related to medical devices can have serious consequences for consumers. Defects in medical devices, such as artificial hips and pacemakers, have caused severe patient injuries and deaths. In 2006, FDA reported 116,086 device-related injuries, 96,485 malfunctions, and 2,830 deaths; an analysis by the National Research Center for Women & Families claims there were 4,556 device-related deaths in 2009. Reports published in 2009 through 2011—by the Government Accountability Office (GAO), the Department of Health and Human Services Office of the Inspector General and the Institute of Medicine—have voiced concerns about FDA's device review process. In 2009 and 2011 GAO included FDA's oversight of medical products on the GAO list of high-risk areas. FDA has conducted internal reviews as well and is implementing changes.

INTRODUCTION

Medical device regulation is complex, in part because of the wide variety of items that are categorized as medical devices. They may be simple tools used during medical examinations, such as tongue depressors and thermometers, or high-tech life-saving implants like heart valves and coronary stents. The medical device market has been characterized as including eight industry sectors: surgical and medical instrument manufacturing, surgical appliance and supplies, in vitro diagnostic products (IVDs, or laboratory tests), electromedical and electrotherapeutic apparatus, irradiation apparatus, dental equipment and supplies, ophthalmic goods, and dental laboratories.[1]

The federal agency primarily responsible for regulating medical devices is the Food and Drug Administration (FDA)—an agency within the Department of Health and Human Services (HHS). A manufacturer must receive FDA permission before its device can be legally marketed in the United States. FDA's Center for Devices and Radiological Health (CDRH) is primarily responsible for medical device review. Another center, the Center for Biologics Evaluation and Research (CBER), regulates devices associated with blood collection and processing procedures, cellular products and tissues.[2]

CDRH activities are funded through a combination of public money (i.e., direct FDA appropriations from Congress) and private money (i.e., user fees collected from device manufacturers) which together comprise FDA's total.[3] User fees may be used only to support product review activities, not other CDRH activities. User fees account for 33% of FDA's total FY2011 program level and 15% of CDRH's program level, which is $378 million in FY2011 including $56 million in user fees.[4] Congress has reauthorized in five-year increments FDA collection of medical device user fees; authority will expire on October 1, 2012 under the terms of the Medical Device User Fee Act of 2007 (MDUFA), Title II of the FDA Amendments Act of 2007 (FDAAA, P.L. 110-85).

Congress has historically been interested in balancing the goals of allowing consumers to have access, as quickly as possible, to new and improved medical devices with preventing devices that are not safe and effective from entering or remaining on the market. The goals of device availability and device safety may exert opposite pulls, with implications for consumers, the health care system, and the economy.

Investment in medical device development reportedly reached a high of $3.690 billion in 2007. Investment has slowed somewhat to $2.380 billion in 2010, and $1.510 billion in the first two quarters of 2011.[5] According to one report, the medical technology industry is a "vibrant and growing contributor to the U.S. economy, generating US$197 billion in revenue and employing over a half million workers in 2009 alone."[6] "Medical technology industry" includes "medical device, diagnostic, drug delivery and analytic/life science tool companies but excludes distributors and service providers" such as contract research or contract manufacturing organizations.[7] Another analysis found that "32 of the 46 medical technology companies with more than $1 billion in annual revenue are based in the United States."[8] Although the largest companies dominate the market for devices in terms of sales, it is often the small device companies that make a significant contribution to early innovation. Small companies may partner with larger companies to bring products to market if they lack access to the capital and resources to conduct clinical trials and navigate regulatory and reimbursement hurdles.

Manufacturers make decisions about pursuing new devices based in part on the cost of their development. Additional regulatory requirements may escalate these costs, while other incentives, such as tax breaks or market exclusivity extensions, may diminish them. If the device development cost is too high, the eventual result may be that consumers are denied access because new products are not developed or brought to market. Access problems have led to proposals for, and the enactment of, incentives to develop medical devices for rare diseases and pediatric populations. However, if the regulation and oversight of device development are not stringent enough, unsafe or ineffective products may reach the market and cause harm to consumers.

Problems related to medical devices can have serious consequences for consumers. Defects in medical devices, such as artificial hips, pacemakers, defibrillators, and stents, have caused severe patient injuries and deaths.[9] In 2006, FDA reported 116,086 device-related injuries, 96,485 malfunctions, and

2,830 deaths; a more recent independent analysis claims there were 4,556 device-related deaths in 2009.[10] Consequences such as these have raised questions as to whether adequate enforcement tools, resources, and processes are in place to ensure that marketed devices are safe. Reports by the Government Accountability Office (GAO), the Department of Health and Human Services Office of the Inspector General, and the Institute of Medicine (IOM) have voiced concerns about FDA's device review process.[11] In 2009 and in 2011 GAO included FDA's oversight of medical products on the GAO list of high-risk areas.[12]

This report provides a description of FDA's medical device review process divided into two parts: premarket requirements and postmarket requirements. **Appendix A** provides a brief history of laws governing medical device regulation and **Appendix B** provides a table of acronyms used in the report.

THE MEDICAL DEVICE REVIEW PROCESS: PREMARKET REQUIREMENTS

FDA requires all medical product manufacturers to register their facilities, list their devices with the agency, and follow general controls requirements.[13] FDA classifies devices according to the risk they pose to consumers. Many medical devices, such as plastic bandages and ice bags, present only minimal risk and can be legally marketed upon registration alone. These low-risk devices are deemed *exempt* from premarket review and manufacturers need not submit an application to FDA prior to marketing.[14] In contrast, most moderate- and high-risk devices must obtain the agency's permission prior to marketing. FDA grants this permission when a manufacturer meets regulatory premarket requirements and agrees to any necessary postmarket requirements which vary according to the risk that a device presents.[15]

PMA vs. 510(k)

There is a fundamental difference between the PMA and 510(k) pathways. In a PMA review, FDA determines if the device is reasonably safe and effective for its intended use. In a 510(k) review, FDA determines if the device is substantially equivalent to another device whose safety and effectiveness may never have been assessed.

There are two paths that manufacturers can use to bring their moderate- and high-risk devices to market with FDA's permission. One path consists of conducting clinical studies, submitting a *premarket approval* (PMA) application and requires evidence providing reasonable assurance that the device is safe and effective.[16] The PMA process is generally used for novel and high-risk devices and is typically lengthy and expensive. It results in a type of FDA permission called *approval.*

The other path involves submitting a *510(k) notification* demonstrating that the device is *substantially equivalent* to a device already on the market (*a predicate device*) that does not require a PMA.[17] The 510(k) process is unique to medical devices and results in FDA *clearance*. Substantial equivalence is determined by comparing the performance characteristics of a new device with those of a predicate device. To be considered substantially equivalent, the new device must have the same intended use and technological characteristics as the predicate; clinical data demonstrating safety and effectiveness are usually not required. The manufacturer selects the predicate device to compare with its new device. However, FDA has the ultimate discretion in determining whether a comparison is appropriate.

According to a 2009 GAO report, of the more than 50,000 devices that were listed by manufacturers with FDA from FY2003 through FY2007, about 67% were exempt from premarket review; the remainder entered the market via the 510(k) process (31%), the PMA process (1%) or via other means.[18]

Device Classification

Under the terms of the Medical Device Amendments of 1976 (MDA, P.L. 94-295), FDA classified all medical devices that were on the market at the time of enactment—the *preamendment* devices—into one of three classes. Congress provided definitions for the three classes—Class I, Class II, Class III—based on the risk (low-, moderate-, and high-risk respectively) to patients posed by the devices.[19] Examples of each class are listed in **Table 1**. Device classification determines the type of regulatory requirements that a manufacturer must follow. Regulatory requirements for each class are described below in more detail. *General controls*, the minimum regulations that apply to all FDA regulated medical devices, include five elements:[20]

- *establishment registration*—such as manufacturers, distributors, repackagers and relabelers, and foreign firms;[21]
- *device listing*—listing with FDA of all devices to be marketed;
- good manufacturing practices (GMP)—manufacturing of devices in accordance with the Quality Systems Regulation (QSR);[22]
- *labeling*—labeling of devices or in vitro diagnostic products;[23] and
- *premarket notification*—submission to FDA of a premarket notification 510(k).

Class I devices are those under current law for which general controls "are sufficient to provide reasonable assurance of the safety and effectiveness of the device."[24] Many Class I devices are *exempt* from the premarket notification and/or the QSR requirements, though they still have to comply with the other general controls. A device is exempt if FDA determines that it presents a low risk of illness or injury to patients.[25]

Table 1. Medical Device Classification

Device Classification	Examples	Safety / Effectiveness Controls	Required Submission
Class I	elastic bandages, examination gloves, and hand-held surgical instruments	General Controls	• *Registration only* unless 510(k) specifically required
Class II	powered wheelchairs, infusion pumps, and surgical drapes	General Controls & Special Controls	• *510(k) clearance* unless exempt • *IDE possible*
Class III	heart valves, silicone gel-filled breast implants, and implanted cerebella stimulators	General Controls & Premarket Approval	• *PMA approval* • *IDE probable*
	metal-on-metal hip joint, certain dental implants	General Controls	• *510(k) clearance*

Source: FDA, Overview of Medical Device Regulation, General and Special Controls, at http://www.fda.gov/MedicalDevices/DeviceRegulationandGuidance/Overview/GeneralandSpecialControls/default.htm.

Note: IDE means investigational device exemption.

Class II devices are those under current law "which cannot be classified as class I because the general controls by themselves are insufficient to provide reasonable assurance of safety and effectiveness of the device."[26] Class II includes devices that pose a moderate risk to patients, and may include new devices for which information or *special controls* are available to reduce or mitigate risk. Special controls may include special labeling requirements, mandatory performance standards, and postmarket surveillance. Currently "15% of all device types classified in Class II are subject to special controls."[27] Although most Class II devices require premarket notification via the 510(k) process, a few are exempt by regulation.[28]

Class III devices are those under current law which "cannot be classified as a class I device because insufficient information exists to determine that the application of general controls are sufficient to provide reasonable assurance of the safety and effectiveness of the device," and "cannot be classified as a class II device because insufficient information exists to determine that the special controls ... would provide reasonable assurance of [their] safety and effectiveness," and are "purported or represented to be for a use in supporting or sustaining human life or for a use which is of substantial importance in preventing impairment of human health," or present "a potential unreasonable risk of illness or injury, [are] to be subject ... to premarket approval to provide reasonable assurance of [their] safety and effectiveness."[29]

In other words, general and/or special controls are not sufficient to assure safe and effective use of a Class III device. Class III includes devices which are life-supporting or life-sustaining, and devices which present a high or potentially unreasonable risk of illness or injury to a patient. New devices that are not classified as Class I or II by another means, are automatically designated as Class III unless the manufacturer files a request or petition for reclassification.[30]

Although most Class III devices require *premarket approval* (PMA), some Class III devices may be cleared via the 510(k) process. In fact, during the first 10 years following enactment of MDA, over 80% of postamendment Class III devices entered the market on the basis of 510(k) submissions showing substantial equivalence to preamendment devices.[31] According to FDA, these are "postamendment (i.e., introduced to the U.S. market after May 28, 1976) Class III devices which are substantially equivalent to preamendment (i.e., introduced to the U.S. market before May 28, 1976) Class III devices and for which the regulation calling for the premarket approval application has not been published in 21 CFR."[32] FDA explains the situation as follows:

> When FDA's medical device regulation program began in the late 1970s, FDA regulated over 100 Class III device types through the 510(k) program. The intent was that FDA's regulation would be temporary and that over time, FDA would decide to reclassify those device types (or regulations) into Class I or II, or to sustain the classification in Class III and call for PMA applications. The process of reclassification is described in FDA's regulations in Section 515 of the Federal Food, Drug and Cosmetic Act. Over the years, FDA has made progress in this original list; however, as of 2009, 26 medical device regulations remained in this transitional state awaiting final classification.[33]

At the time that the MDA of 1976 was drafted, "relatively few medical devices were permanently implanted or intended to sustain life. The 510(k) process was specifically intended for devices with less need for scientific scrutiny, such as surgical gloves and hearing aids."[34] Over time, FDA's 510(k) review process was "challenged as new devices changed more dramatically and became more complex."[35]

Examples of Class III devices that are still regulated via the 510(k) program include the metal-on-metal hip joint, certain dental implants, automated external defibrillator, electroconvulsive therapy device, pedicle screw spinal system, intra-aortic balloon and control system, and several device types related to pacemakers.[36] In late 2009, FDA implemented the 515 Program Initiative "to facilitate the final adjudication of these remaining Class III device types."[37]

Medical Device Marketing Applications

As stated above, in general, before a non-exempt medical device may be legally marketed, a manufacturer must submit to FDA either: a PMA application, and the agency *approves* the device; or, a 510(k) notification, and the agency *clears* the device. FDA makes its determination—either approval or clearance—based on information the manufacturer submits. The information that is required—in other words, the type of marketing application the manufacturer must make (if any)—is determined based on the *risk* that the device poses, if used according to the manufacturer's instructions. FDA typically evaluates more than 4,000 510(k) notifications and about 40 original PMA applications each year.[38]

The Food and Drug Administration Modernization Act of 1997 (FDAMA; P.L. 105-115) gave FDA the authority to establish procedures for meeting with manufacturers prior to preparing a submission.[39] The procedures aim to speed the review process by giving FDA and a manufacturer the opportunity to address questions and concerns about the device and/or the planned studies that will be used to support the marketing application before the studies are initiated and the application is submitted. Requests for these meetings have doubled over the past five years according to testimony by CDRH Director Jeffrey Shuren at a November 2011 Senate hearing.[40]

Generally speaking, under the Federal Food, Drug and Cosmetic Act (FFDCA), manufacturers

- are prohibited from selling an adulterated product;[41]
- are prohibited from misbranding a product;[42]
- must register their facility with FDA and list all of the medical devices that they produce or process (and a fee is now required under the terms of FDAAA);
- must file the appropriate premarket submission with the agency at least 90 days before introducing a *non-exempt* device onto the market; and
- must report to FDA any incident that they are aware of that suggests that their device may have caused or contributed to a death or serious injury.

Under the terms of MDUFA (Title II of FDAAA), manufacturers must pay a fee for most types of submissions. In 2010, FDA charged $217,787 in user fees to review a PMA ($54,447 for smaller companies) and $4,007 to review a 510(k) submission ($2,004 for small companies).[43] GAO found that in 2005, the average cost for FDA to review a PMA was $870,000 and the average cost to review a 510(k) submission was $18,200.[44] According to CDRH Director Jeffrey Shuren, user fees collected under MDUFA "fund only about 20% of the device review program;" in contrast, users fees collected under the Prescription Drug User Fee Act (PDUFA) "account for about two-thirds of the drug review program's budget."[45]

510(k) Notification

In general, a 510(k) submission is required for a moderate-risk medical device that is not non-exempt from premarket review. A 510(k) could also be used for currently marketed devices for which the manufacturer seeks a new indication (e.g., a new population, such as pediatric use, or a new disease or condition), or for which the manufacturer has changed the design or technical characteristics such that the change may affect the performance characteristics of the device.

Between 1996 and 2009, more than 80% of the devices cleared by FDA using 510(k) notification were Class II devices, about 10% were Class I and less than 5% were Class III.[46] A 2009 GAO report found that 25% of the 10,670 Class II devices cleared by FDA in FY2003 through FY2007 were either implantable, life sustaining or presented significant risk to the health, safety, or welfare of the patient.[47] The agency cleared about 90% of 510(k) submissions reviewed during FY2003 through FY2007.[48]

As noted previously, the standard for clearance of a traditional 510(k) is substantial equivalence with a predicate device. A predicate device can be one of two things. It can be a previously cleared Class I or II device that does not require a PMA. It can also be preamendment Class III for which the agency has not issued regulations requiring a PMA. (PMAs, which are more rigorous submissions than 510(k)s, are discussed in the "Premarket Approval (PMA)" section.)

A manufacturer may choose one of three types of 510(k) submissions for premarket clearance: traditional, special, or abbreviated.[49] A study of 510(k) submissions between 1996 and 2009 found that about 80% were traditional, 16% were special, and 3% were abbreviated.[50] For novel devices without a predicate, there is another alternative called the de novo 510(k) process.

In a traditional 510(k), the manufacturer submits information about the performance of the device under specific conditions of use. It also contains information about the design of the device, characteristics of device components, representations of packaging and labeling, a description and summary of the non-clinical and clinical studies that were done to support the device performance characteristics, a description of means by which users can assess the quality of the device, and information about any computer software or additional or special equipment needed. Several administrative forms are also required.[51]

Most of the studies supporting a 510(k) submission are not clinical studies. Substantial equivalence, in many cases, means only that the device performs in a similar fashion to the predicate under a similar set of circumstances. As a result, many devices never have to demonstrate safety and effectiveness through clinical studies.

2011 IOM Report on 510(k) Substantial Equivalence

"In practice, the assessment of substantial equivalence generally does not require evidence of safety or effectiveness of a device. Unlike the premarket approval (PMA) process, by law the 510(k) process, with some exceptions [see SMDA 1990], focuses solely on the determination of a device's substantial equivalence to a predicate device. According to the FDA and the Supreme Court, when the FDA finds a device substantially equivalent to a predicate device, it has done no more than find that the new device is as safe and effective as the predicate. It is important to note that devices on the market before the enactment of the 1976 Medical Device Amendments (MDA)—the origin of all predicate devices for the 510(k) process—have never been systematically assessed to determine their safety and effectiveness. Because the preamendment device to which equivalence was established was not itself reviewed for safety or effectiveness, the committee found that clearance of a 510(k) submission was not a determination that the cleared device was safe or effective." See p. 154.

In addition to not requiring clinical studies, three other characteristics of the 510(k) process make it much less rigorous than the PMA process: (1) premarket inspections of how devices were manufactured are generally not required by FDA; (2) postmarket studies are not required by FDA as a condition of clearance; and, (3) FDA has limited authority to rescind or withdraw clearance if a 510(k) device is found to be unsafe or ineffective.[52]

FDA may take any of the following actions on a 510(k) after conducting its review:

- find the device substantially equivalent to the predicate and issue a clearance letter;
- find the device not substantially equivalent (NSE) and issue an NSE letter prohibiting marketing;
- determine that the device is exempt from a 510(k) submission;
- request additional information (with the final clearance decision pending review of that information).[53]

A manufacturer generally has 30 days to provide any additional information, or FDA may issue a notice of withdrawal of the application.[54] The manufacturer may, at any time, withdraw its 510(k). FDA has 90 days to review a traditional 510(k).[55]

Abbreviated and special 510(k)s were new approaches to premarket notification that came from FDAMA. These approaches were intended to streamline and expedite FDA's review for routine submissions meeting certain qualifications, thus leaving reviewer time for more complicated submissions.

An abbreviated 510(k) uses guidance documents developed by FDA to communicate regulatory and scientific expectations to industry. Guidance documents have been prepared for many different kinds of devices, and are available on FDA's website. All guidance documents are developed in accordance with Good Guidance Practices (GGP), and many with public participation or opportunities for public comment.[56] In addition to issuing guidance documents, FDA can either develop performance or consensus standards or 'recognize' those developed by outside parties.[57] In an abbreviated 510(k), the manufacturer describes what guidance document, special control, or performance standard was used, and how it was used to assess performance of their device. Other minimum required elements are the product description, representative labeling, and a summary of the performance characteristics. FDA typically reviews an abbreviated 510(k) in 60 days.

A special 510(k) may be used for a modification to a device that has already been cleared; it typically uses the design control[58] requirement of the Quality System Regulation (QSR). The QSR describes the good manufacturing practice (GMP) requirements for medical devices.[59] The special 510(k) allows the manufacturer to declare conformance to design controls without providing the data. This type of submission references the original 510(k) number, and contains information about the design control requirements. FDA aims to review most special 510(k)s in 30 days.

Under the FFDCA, novel devices lacking a legally marketed predicate are automatically designated Class III. FDAMA amended FFDCA Section 513(f) to allow FDA to establish a new, expedited mechanism for reclassifying these devices based on risk, thus reducing the regulatory burden on manufacturers. The de novo 510(k), though requiring more data than a traditional 510(k), often requires less information than a premarket approval (PMA) application.

In a de novo 510(k) process, the manufacturer submits a traditional 510(k) for its device. However, because there is no predicate device or classification, the agency will return a decision of not substantially equivalent. Within 30 days, the manufacturer submits a petition requesting reclassification of its device into Class II or I, as appropriate. Within 60 days, FDA will render a decision classifying the device according to criteria in FFDCA Section 513(a)(1). With approval, FDA issues a regulation that classifies the device. If the device is Class II, a special controls guidance document is also developed that then allows subsequent manufacturers to submit either traditional or abbreviated 510(k)s.[60] On September 30, 2011, FDA released draft guidance designed to further streamline the de novo review process.[61]

Premarket Approval (PMA)

A PMA is the most stringent type of device marketing application required by FDA for new and/or high-risk devices. PMA approval is based on a determination by FDA that the application contains sufficient valid scientific evidence to assure that the device is safe and effective for its intended use(s).[62] In contrast to a 510(k), PMAs generally require some clinical data prior to gaining approval.[63] All clinical evaluations of investigational devices (unless exempt) must have an investigational device exemption (IDE) before the study is initiated.[64] An IDE allows an unapproved device (most commonly an invasive or life-sustaining device) to be used in a clinical study to collect the data required to support a PMA submission.[65] The IDE permits a device to be shipped lawfully for investigation of the device without requiring that the manufacturer comply with other requirements of the FFDCA, such as registration and listing. In August and in November 2011 FDA released new draft guidance intended to ensure the quality of clinical trials and streamline the IDE process by clarifying the criteria for approving clinical trials.[66] All clinical studies must also receive prior approval by an institutional review board (IRB).[67]

A PMA must contain (among other things) the following information:

- summaries of non-clinical and clinical data supporting the intended use and performance characteristics;
- detailed information on the device design and device components;
- instructions for use;
- representations of packaging and labeling;
- a description of means by which users can assess the quality of the device;
- information about computer software or additional or special equipment;
- literature about the disease and the similar devices; and,
- information on the manufacturing process.

Approval is based not only on the strength of the scientific data, but also on inspection of the manufacturing facility to assure that the facility and the manufacturing process are in compliance with the quality systems regulations (QSR).[68] FDAMA made it easier for manufacturers to submit the required sections of a PMA in a serial fashion as data are available ("modular PMA").

When a PMA is first received, FDA has 45 days to make sure the application is administratively complete. If not, the application is returned. If the application is complete, it is formally filed by FDA. The agency then has 75 days to complete the initial review and determine whether an advisory committee meeting will be necessary.

Advisory committees can be convened to make recommendations on any scientific or policy matter before FDA.[69] They are comprised of scientific, medical, and statistical experts, and industry and consumer representatives. An advisory committee meeting allows interested persons to present information and views at a public hearing.[70] FDA typically accepts advisory committee recommendations for an application (approvable, approvable with conditions, or non-approvable). However, there have been cases where FDA's decision has not been consistent with the committee's recommendation. CDRH will hold joint advisory committee meetings with other centers where necessary.

After FDA notifies the applicant that the PMA has been approved or denied, a notice may be published on the Internet announcing the data on which the decision is based and providing interested persons an opportunity to petition FDA within 30 days for reconsideration of the decision. Though FDA regulations allow 180 days to review the PMA and make a determination, total review time can be much longer.[71] MDUFA performance goals have been established to reduce the review time for PMAs.[72]

THE MEDICAL DEVICE REVIEW PROCESS: POST-MARKET REQUIREMENTS

Once approved or cleared for marketing, manufacturers of medical devices must comply with various regulations on labeling and advertising, manufacturing, postmarketing surveillance, device tracking, and adverse event reporting. This section describes those requirements and the Sentinel Initiative and the unique device identification (UDI) system, which are both under development, as well as CDRH compliance and enforcement actions.

Labeling

Like drugs and biological products, all FDA approved or cleared medical devices are required to be labeled in a way that informs a user of how to use the device. The FFDCA defines a "label" as a "display of written, printed, or graphic matter upon the immediate container of any article."[73] "Labeling" is defined as "all labels and other written, printed, or graphic matter upon any article or any of its containers or wrappers, or accompanying such article" at any time while a device is held for sale after shipment or delivery for shipment in interstate commerce.[74] The term "accompanying" is interpreted to mean more than physical association with the product; it extends to posters, tags, pamphlets, circulars, booklets, brochures, instruction books, direction sheets, fillers, webpages, etc. Accompanying can also include labeling that is connected with the device after shipment or delivery for shipment in interstate commerce. According to an appellate court decision, "most, if not all advertising, is labeling. The term 'labeling' is defined in the FFDCA as including all printed matter accompanying any article. Congress did not, and we cannot, exclude from the definition printed matter which constitutes advertising."[75] All devices must conform to the general labeling requirements.[76] Certain devices require specific labeling which may include not only package labeling, but informational literature, patient release forms, performance testing, and/or specific tolerances or prohibitions on certain ingredients.[77]

A section of the QSR also has an impact on various aspects of labeling.[78] The QSR regulation applies to the application of labeling to ensure legibility under normal conditions of use over the expected life of the device and also applies to inspection, handling, storage, and distribution of labeling. FDA considers a device to be adulterated if these requirements are not met. These requirements do not apply to the adequacy of labeling content, except to make sure the content meets labeling specifications contained in the device master record. However, failure to comply with GMP requirements, such as proofreading and change control, could result in labeling content errors. In such cases, the device could be misbranded and/or adulterated.

Manufacturing

Like drug manufacturers, medical device manufacturers must produce their devices in accordance with Good Manufacturing Practice (GMP). The

GMP requirements for devices are described in the QSR.[79] The QSRs require that domestic or foreign manufacturers have a quality system for the design, manufacture, packaging, labeling, storage, installation, and servicing of non-exempt finished medical devices intended for commercial distribution in the United States. The regulation requires that various specifications and controls be established for devices; that devices be designed and manufactured under a quality system to meet these specifications; that finished devices meet these specifications; that devices be correctly installed, checked and serviced; that quality data be analyzed to identify and correct quality problems; and thatcomplaints be processed. FDA monitors device problem data and inspects the operations and records of device developers and manufacturers to determine compliance with the GMP requirements.[80] Though FDA has identified in QSR the essential elements that a quality system should have, manufacturers have a great deal of leeway to design quality systems that best cover nuances of their devices and the means of producing them.

Postmarketing Surveillance

The 2011 IOM report states that because "it is not possible to create a premarket review process that could completely ensure the safety of all devices before they enter the market, a strong surveillance system that monitors the safety of medical devices is essential. The identification of problems associated with a medical device can be an opportunity for various corrective actions."[81] Such actions might include changing the device labeling and instructions for use, improving user training, or removal of the device from the market if appropriate. While the term postmarketing surveillance refers to a wide range of programs, the term postmarket surveillance refers to a specific activity defined in law.[82]

Postmarket Surveillance

For certain devices introduced into interstate commerce after January 1, 1991, manufacturers must conduct postmarket surveillance studies, once their device is approved or cleared for marketing, in order to gather safety and efficacy data. This requirement applies to devices that

- are permanent implants, the failure of which may cause serious adverse health consequences or death;
- are intended for use in supporting or sustaining human life; or

- present a potential serious risk to human health.

FDA may require postmarket surveillance for other devices if deemed necessary to protect the public health. The primary objective of postmarket surveillance is to study the performance of the device after clearance or approval as it is used in the population for which it is intended—and to discover cases of device failure and its attendant impact on the patient. Manufacturers may receive notification that their device is subject to postmarket surveillance when FDA files (i.e., accepts) the submission, and again when a final decision is made. If notified, manufacturers must submit a plan for postmarket surveillance to FDA for approval within 30 days of introducing their device into interstate commerce. MDUFA authorized the appropriation of $25 million per year for Postmarket Studies and Surveillance.[83]

Adverse Event Reporting

The Safe Medical Devices Act of 1990 (SMDA, P.L. 101-629) required FDA to establish a system for monitoring and tracking serious adverse events that resulted from the use or misuse of medical devices.[84] The Medical Device Reporting (MDR) regulation is the mechanism that FDA and manufacturers use to identify and monitor significant adverse events involving medical devices, so that problems are detected and corrected in a timely manner.[85]

Device manufacturers are required to report to FDA (1) within 30 calendar days of acquiring information that reasonably suggests one of their devices may have caused or contributed to a death, serious injury, or malfunction and (2) within 5 working days if an event requires action other than routine maintenance or service to prevent a public health issue.[86] User facilities, such as hospitals and nursing homes, are also required to report deaths to both the manufacturer, if known, and FDA within 10 working days.[87] User facilities must report serious injuries to the manufacturers (or FDA if the manufacturer is unknown) within 10 working days.[88] User facilities must also submit annual reports to FDA of all adverse event reports sent to manufacturers or FDA in the past year.[89]

In August 2009, FDA published notice of a proposed rule, and a related draft guidance document, that would require manufacturers to submit MDRs to the agency in an electronic format.[90] According to FDA, the proposed regulatory changes would provide the agency with a more efficient data entry process that would allow for timely access to medical device adverse event information and identification of emerging public health issues. The device industry requested a longer timeframe to implement the changes.

An October 2009 HHS Office of Inspector General report raised a number of questions about adverse event reporting for medical devices.[91] The report found that CDRH does not consistently use adverse event reporting and made several recommendations about how it could better do so.

Medical Device Tracking

Manufacturers are required to track certain devices from their manufacture through the distribution chain when they receive an order from FDA to implement a tracking system for a certain type of device.[92] The purpose of device tracking is to ensure that manufacturers of these devices can locate them quickly once in commercial distribution if needed to facilitate notifications and recalls in the case of serious risks to health presented by the devices. FDA may issue a tracking order for any Class II or Class III device:

- the failure of which would be reasonably likely to have serious adverse health consequences;
- which is intended to be implanted in the human body for more than one year; or
- which is intended to be a life sustaining or life supporting device used outside a device user facility.[93]

FDA has issued orders to track 13 implantable devices (including silicone gel-filled breast implants, various joint prostheses, implantable pacemakers, implantable defibrillator, mechanical heart valves, and implantable infusion pumps) and four other devices that are used outside a device user facility.[94]

The Sentinel Initiative

Section 905 of FDAAA mandated that FDA create an active postmarket risk identification system.[95] Although the FDAAA language is focused on monitoring drugs, FDA is using its general authority to monitor all FDA-regulated products, including medical devices, after they have reached the market.[96] FDA launched the Sentinel Initiative in May 2008; once completed, it will be called the Sentinel System. FDAAA set goals that the new system must be able to access data on 25 million people by July 2010, a goal which FDA has met, and 100 million people by July 2012.[97] As of January 2011 FDA has the capacity to access data from the electronic health records of more than 60 million people.[98]

FDA is collaborating with institutions throughout the United States, including academic medical centers, healthcare systems and health insurance companies, who act as data partners in the system. Additional collaborators will include patient and healthcare professional advocacy groups, academic institutions and the medical products industry. As an example of data applicable to medical devices, "one Sentinel-related project identified, described, and evaluated potential US orthopedic-implant registries that could participate in the creation of a national network of such registries as part of the Sentinel Initiative. Data related to medical devices include rates of selected outcomes (for example, myocardial infarction and stroke), rates of infection, and rates of implant revision and reintervention."[99] According to FDA, the Sentinel Initiative aims to develop and implement a proactive system that will complement existing systems that the agency has in place to track reports of adverse events linked to the use of its regulated products.[100]

Unique Device Identification

A provision in FDAAA requires the HHS Secretary to promulgate regulations establishing a unique device identification (UDI) system.[101] When implemented, this new system will require

- the label of a device to bear a unique identifier, unless an alternative location is specified by FDA or unless an exception is made for a particular device or group of devices;
- the unique identifier to be able to identify the device through distribution and use; and
- the unique identifier to include the lot or serial number if specified by FDA.

According to FDA, "incorporation of UDI into various health-related databases will greatly facilitate many important public health-related activities including: reducing medical errors; reporting and assessing device-related adverse events and product problems; tracking of recalls; assessing patient-centered outcomes and the risk/benefit profile of medical devices in large segments of the U.S. population; and, providing an easily accessible source of device identification information to patients and health care professionals."[102]

CDRH indicated in its FY2010 Strategic Priorities that the UDI system will be implemented by September 30, 2013.[103] UDI will be implemented in three phases: Class III devices will need to be in compliance within one year after the final rule is published, Class II at three years and Class I at five years after the final rule.[104] FDA has held a number of public meetings and workshops with stakeholders to discuss the adoption, implementation, and use of a UDI system. The agency has posted on its website information about these meetings as well as a number of reports on the use of UDI for medical devices.[105]

FDA has been working with the Global Harmonization Task Force (GHTF) to foster international harmonization in the regulation of medical devices through the development of non-binding guidance documents.[106] The GHTF is a voluntary international group of representatives from medical device regulatory authorities and trade associations from Europe, the United States, Canada, Japan and Australia. In September 2011 the GHTF published its final document on UDI for medical devices.[107]

Compliance and Enforcement

Compliance requirements apply to both the premarket approval process and postmarket surveillance. When a problem arises with a product regulated by FDA, the agency can take a number of actions to protect the public health. Initially, the agency tries to work with the manufacturer to correct the problem on a voluntary basis. If that fails, legal remedies may be taken, such as: asking the manufacturer to recall a product, having federal marshals seize products, or detaining imports at the port of entry until problems are corrected. If warranted, FDA can ask the courts to issue injunctions or prosecute individual company officers that deliberately violate the law. When warranted, criminal penalties, including prison sentences, may be sought.

Section 516 of the FFDCA gives FDA the authority to ban devices that present substantial deception or unreasonable and substantial risk of illness or injury. Section 518 enables FDA to require manufacturers or other appropriate individuals to notify all health professionals who prescribe or use the device and any other person (including manufacturers, importers, distributors, retailers, and device users) of any health risks resulting from the use of a violative device, so that these risks may be reduced or eliminated. This section also gives consumers a procedure for economic redress when they have been sold defective medical devices that present unreasonable risks. Section 519 of the act authorized FDA to promulgate regulations requiring manufacturers, importers, and distributors of devices to maintain records and reports to assure that devices are not adulterated or misbranded. Section 520(e) authorizes FDA to restrict the sale, distribution, or use of a device if there cannot otherwise be reasonable assurance of its safety and effectiveness. A restricted device can only be sold on oral or written authorization by a licensed practitioner or under conditions specified by regulation.

Inspection

Each FDA center has an Office of Compliance (OC) that ensures compliance with regulations while pre- or postmarket studies are being undertaken, with manufacturing requirements, and with labeling requirements. The objectives of CDRH's OC's Bioresearch Monitoring (BIMO) program are to ensure the quality and integrity of data and information submitted in support of IDE, PMA, and 510(k) submissions and to ensure that human subjects taking part in investigations are protected from undue hazard or risk. This is achieved through audits of clinical data contained in PMAs prior to approval, data audits of IDE and 510(k) submissions, inspections of IRBs and nonclinical laboratories, and enforcement of the prohibitions against promotion, marketing, or commercialization of investigational devices. Any establishment where devices are manufactured, processed, packed, installed, used, or implanted or where records of results from use of devices are kept, can be subject to inspection. (See **Table 2.**)

The OC also reviews the quality system design and manufacturing information in the PMA submission to determine whether the manufacturer has described the processes in sufficient detail and to make a preliminary determination of whether the manufacturer meets the QSR. If the manufacturer has provided an adequate description of the design and manufacturing process, a preapproval inspection can be initiated. Inspection is to include an assessment of the manufacturer's capability to design and manufacture the device as claimed in the PMA and confirm that the quality system is in compliance with the QSR. Postapproval inspections can be conducted within 8 to 12 months of approval of the PMA submission. The inspection is to primarily focus on any changes that may have been made in the device design, manufacturing process, or quality systems.

Table 2. CDRH, FDA Foreign and Domestic Inspections, FY2004–FY2010

FY	2004	2005	2006	2007	2008	2009	2010
Number of Inspections	2,936	2,694	2,691	2,495	2,353	2,550	3,174

Source: FDA Center for Devices and Radiological Health, Office of Compliance, Division of Risk Management Operations based on Center Ad Hoc Reporting System inspection data.

The compliance offices work closely with the Office of Regulatory Affairs (ORA),[108] which operates in the field to regulate almost 124,000 business establishments that annually produce, warehouse, import and transport $1 trillion worth of medical products. Consumer safety officers (CSOs) and inspectors typically have conducted about 22,000 domestic and foreign inspections a year to ensure that regulated products meet the agency's standards. CSOs also monitor clinical trials. Scientists in ORA's 13 laboratories typically have analyzed more than 41,000 product samples each year to determine their adherence to FDA's standards.

Warning Letter

A warning letter is a written communication from FDA notifying a responsible individual, manufacturer, or facility that the agency considers one or more products, practices, processes, or other activities to be in violation of the laws that FDA enforces. The warning letter informs the recipient that failure to take appropriate and prompt action to correct and prevent any future repeat of the violations could result in an administrative or regulatory action. Although serious noncompliance is often a catalyst for issuance of a warning letter, the warning letter is informal and advisory.[109] (See **Table 3.**)

Table 3. CDRH Warning Letters Issued, FY2000–FY2010

FY	2000	2001	2002	2003	2004	2005	2006	2007	2008	2009	2010
Number of Letters	528	498	285	205	198	182	154	155	152	136	204

Source: FDA Center for Devices and Radiological Health, Office of Compliance, Division of Risk Management Operations based on Office of Regulatory Affairs Case Management System warning letter data.

Product Recall

A recall is a method of removing or correcting products that FDA considers are in violation of the law.[110] Medical device recalls are usually conducted voluntarily by the manufacturer after negotiation with FDA.[111] Manufacturers (including refurbishers and reconditioners) and importers are required to report to FDA any correction or removal of a medical device that is undertaken to reduce a health risk posed by the device.[112] A recall may be a total market withdrawal or may be of a portion of product (such as a single lot). In rare instances, where the manufacturer or importer fails to voluntarily recall a device that is a risk to health, FDA may issue a recall order to the manufacturer.[113]

When a recall is initiated, FDA performs an evaluation of the health hazard presented taking into account the following factors, among others:

- Whether any disease or injuries have occurred from the use of the product;
- Whether any existing conditions could contribute to a clinical situation that could expose humans or animals to a health hazard;
- Assessment of hazard to various populations (e.g., children, surgical patients, pets, livestock) who would be exposed to the product;
- Assessment of the degree of seriousness of the health hazard to which the populations at risk would be exposed;
- Assessment of the likelihood of occurrence of the hazard;
- Assessment of the consequences (immediate or long-range) of the hazard.

Following the health hazard assessment, FDA assigns the recall a classification according to the relative degree of health hazard. *Class I* recalls are the most serious, reserved for situations where there is a reasonable probability that the use of, or exposure to, a product will cause serious adverse health consequences or death. *Class II* recalls are for situations where the use of, or exposure to, a product may cause temporary or medically reversible adverse health consequences or where the probability of serious adverse health consequences is remote. In a *Class III* recall situation, the use of, or exposure to, a product is not likely to cause adverse health consequences. (See **Table 4.**) In addition to a warning letter or recall, FDA may issue a public notification or safety alert (e.g., "Dear Doctor" letter), to warn healthcare providers and consumers of the risk of the device.[114]

Table 4. CDRH Class I, II, and III Product Recalls, FY2004–FY2010

FY	2004	2005	2006	2007	2008	2009	2010
Class I	36	77	76	45	131	219	334
Class II	1,235	1,351	1,252	1,102	2,178	2,222	2,208
Class III	219	170	222	132	163	194	92

Source: FDA Center for Devices and Radiological Health, Office of Compliance, Division of Risk Management Operations based on Center Ad Hoc Reporting System recall data.

APPENDIX A. HISTORY OF LAWS GOVERNING MEDICAL DEVICE REGULATION

The Federal Food, Drug and Cosmetics Act of 1938

The first general federal food and drug law, the *Food and Drugs Act of 1906*, did not contain any provisions to regulate medical device safety or claims made regarding such devices. Strong support for reform developed during the 1930s due to "false therapeutic claims for medical devices [that] were being presented to the public through radio and newspaper advertising."[115] Medical devices came under federal scrutiny when Congress passed the *Federal Food, Drug and Cosmetic Act (FFDCA) of 1938* (P.L. 75-717). The regulatory authority provided to FDA by the 1938 law was "limited to action after a medical device has been offered for introduction into interstate commerce" and only when the device was deemed to be "adulterated or misbranded."[116]

Most of the legitimate devices on the market at the time the 1938 Act became law "were relatively simple items which applied basic science concepts such that experts using them could readily recognize whether the device was functioning properly; the major concern with respect to these devices was assuring truthful labeling."[117] During the first 20 years following enactment of the 1938 law, FDA's activity with respect to medical devices involved protecting the American public from *fraudulent* devices; FDA began to turn its attention to the hazards from *legitimate* devices around 1960.[118]

> The post-war revolution in biomedical technology had resulted in the introduction of a wide variety of sophisticated devices. New developments in the electronic, plastic, metallurgy, and ceramics industries, coupled with progress in design engineering, led to invention of the heart pacemaker, the kidney dialysis machine, defibrillators, cardiac and renal catheters, surgical implants, artificial vessels and heart valves, intensive care monitoring units, and a wide spectrum of other diagnostic and therapeutic devices. Although many lives have been saved or improved by the new discoveries, the potential for harm to consumers has been heightened by the critical medical conditions in which sophisticated modern devices are used and by the complicated technology involved in their manufacture and use. In the search to expand medical knowledge, new experimental approaches have sometimes been tried without adequate premarket clinical testing, quality control in materials selected, or patient consent.[119]

The Dalkon Shield, a contraceptive device introduced in November 1970, is "an example of a legitimate device which was marketed without adequate premarket testing."[120] Other examples include defective cardiac pacemakers and intraocular lenses which, following implantation, caused unusual eye infections resulting in serious vision impairment or the need for removal of the eye.

Congress amended the FFDCA in 1962 to require FDA approval of a new drug application prior to marketing and to require that a new drug be shown to be effective as well as safe. Following these changes, FDA began "to impose rigorous premarket approval of some products that today would be deemed devices." Court decisions in the late 1960s upheld FDA's authority to regulate some medical devices as drugs due in part to the overlapping definitions of drug and device in the 1938 law. FDA classified a number of devices as drugs (contact lenses, injectable silicone, pregnancy-test kits, bone cement), and only such devices were subject to premarket review (prior to 1976). However the approach of classifying devices as a drug was unsuccessful in other court decisions and the need for more comprehensive authority to regulate devices was recognized by the Kennedy, Johnson and Nixon administrations.[121]

The Medical Device Amendments of 1976

The *Medical Device Amendments of 1976* (MDA; P.L. 94-295) was the first major legislation passed to address the review of medical devices. The MDA provided a definition for the term device.[122] It established a number of requirements referred to as *general controls* that applied to all devices.[123] Examples include provisions on adulteration and misbranding, prohibitions on false or misleading advertising, and a requirement to register all medical device manufacturers with FDA. One such provision required manufacturers to notify FDA 90 days prior to the marketing of any new device; if the agency failed to act, marketing could begin. Because this provision is outlined in section 510(k) of the FFDCA, it is often referred to as a "510(k) notification."

The MDA directed FDA to classify, into one of three classes, all medical devices that were on the market at the time of enactment; these are the *preamendment* devices.[124] Congress provided definitions for the three classes—Class I, Class II, Class III—based on the risks to patients posed by the devices. In contrast to the approach taken with pharmaceuticals (all, except generic agents, undergo rigorous premarket review and approval), Congress limited premarket approval to only a small number of devices. "Only the highest-risk category [Class III] would require agency review and approval as a precondition for commercial sale and routine medical use. The other two categories would be subject not to a rigorous review but merely a requirement [510(k)] that the manufacturer of a device notify FDA, at least 90 days before commencing marketing, of its intent to distribute the product commercially."[125] For Class I devices, no additional review was needed once the status of Class I was confirmed; general controls were considered to be sufficient to protect public health. For Class II devices, limited supplemental review would be needed to verify conformity with performance standards if such standards had been established by the agency.[126]

Under MDA, all devices coming to market after enactment were automatically placed in Class III until reclassified; these are the *postamendment* devices. As stated above, Class III medical devices receive more intense scrutiny and require an application for premarket approval (PMA) before the device can be marketed. However, the MDA allowed for the reclassification of a device from one class to another. According to a 2011 IOM report on medical devices:

> The classification and reclassification process did not include any evaluation of the safety or effectiveness of the device types being categorized. Once a device type was assigned to Class III, the FDA was directed to promulgate a regulation calling for manufacturers of devices of that type to submit a [PMA] application. The agency would then (and only then) undertake a review of the safety and effectiveness of the devices. For device types placed into Class I or Class II, there was no mechanism for the systematic review of safety and effectiveness. Congress envisioned instead that the agency would use its postmarketing tools to identify and address issues of lack of safety or lack of effectiveness case by case. Thus, preamendment devices in Class I and II were never subjected to a comprehensive FDA evaluation for safety or effectiveness. The classification process was not completed until 1988.[127]

For postamendment devices, which were automatically placed into Class III, there were two important exceptions:

> The primary exception involved a postamendment device that was substantially equivalent to another device of the same type that either as a preamendment device that had not been classified into any class or was not a preamendment device but had already been classified into Class I or Class II. The FDA permitted manufacturers of postamendment devices to demonstrate substantial equivalence to a preamendment device in Class I

or II as part of the 510(k) submission. An alternative exception provided that the postamendment device would not be in Class III if the FDA, in response to a petition, classified it into Class I or Class II.[128]

The MDA did not provide a definition for the term *substantially equivalent*. The MDA also did not itemize the required contents of a 510(k). Such a notification "need only set forth its proposed intended use or indications for use, the device to which substantial equivalence is claimed, and evidence demonstrating that equivalence."[129]

The Safe Medical Devices Act of 1990

The *Safe Medical Devices Act of 1990* (SMDA; P.L. 101-629) made a number of changes to the law such as providing a definition for the term *substantial equivalence* and revising the definition for Class II. FDA had not promulgated performance standards for most Class II devices. The new law authorized the use of alternative restrictions, called special controls, at the agency's discretion and simplified the process of establishing performance standards for Class II devices. Examples of special controls include special labeling requirements, mandatory performance standards, patient registries and postmarket surveillance.

FDA also had experienced difficulty in promulgating regulations needed to require submission of PMA applications for Class III devices. SMDA authorized FDA to reconsider all the preamendment devices that had been placed in Class III and reclassify some of these devices into Class I or Class II.[130] The purpose was "to reduce the number of device types that needed PMA review."[131] For those devices remaining in Class III, the agency was directed to establish a schedule for promulgation of regulations calling for PMAs of devices that still used the 510(k) notification as an entry to the marketplace.

Under SMDA, FDA must issue a response to a 510(k) submission before marketing of a new device can begin. SMDA allowed for the evaluation of safety and effectiveness data in 510(k) notifications, but only in certain situations. These were limited to cases in which a new device offered different technologic characteristics from the already marketed *premendment or postamendment* (predicate) device.[132] "Because the assessment of substantial equivalence generally did not require evidence of safety or effectiveness of a device and because a preamendment device to which equivalence was established was not itself reviewed for safety or effectiveness, the FDA made clear from the outset that clearance of a 510(k) notification was not a determination that the cleared device was safe or effective. That position was reiterated by the agency numerous times. The US Supreme Court accepted this interpretation in a 1996 opinion."[133]

U.S. Supreme Court 1996 Opinion
Medtronic v. Lohr

"Substantial equivalence determinations provide little protection to the public. These determinations simply compare a post-1976 device to a pre-1976 device to ascertain whether the latter is no more dangerous and no less effective than the earlier device. If the earlier device poses a severe risk or is ineffective, then the latter device may also be risky or ineffective."

Medtronic, Inc. v. Lohr, 518 U.S. 470 (1996).

SMDA established postmarket requirements for medical devices. SMDA required facilities that use medical devices to report to FDA any incident that suggested that a medical device could have caused or contributed to the death, serious illness, or injury of a patient. Manufacturers of certain permanently implanted devices were required to establish methods for tracking the patients who received them and to conduct postmarket surveillance to identify adverse events. The act authorized FDA to carry out certain enforcement actions, such as device product recalls, for products that did not comply with the law.

The Food and Drug Administration Modernization Act of 1997

The *Food and Drug Administration Modernization Act of 1997* (FDAMA; P.L. 105-115) mandated wide-ranging reforms in the regulation of foods, drugs and medical devices by FDA. In general, provisions involving medical devices "were designed to reduce FDA's workload and permit concentration of resources on devices that presented greater potential for harm" and "to limit the FDA's discretion and authority in regulating the device industry" in order to "accelerate the pace of technology transfer."[134]

FDAMA eliminated the 510(k) notification requirement for most Class I devices and some Class II devices. It authorized the creation of a third-party review system of 510(k) submissions for Class I and most Class II devices that still required 510(k) review. It allowed certain new devices (those not substantially equivalent to another device and automatically placed in Class III) to be evaluated for immediate placement in Class I or Class II. This process, called the de novo 510(k), avoids PMA review, must be completed in 60 days, and may be requested by the sponsor.

For substantial equivalence determinations in which the new device has a different technological characteristic, FDAMA requires that FDA "consider the least burdensome means of demonstrating substantial equivalence and request information accordingly."[135] For a medical device using an important breakthrough technology, or which does not have an approved alternative device, priority review of the PMA must be provided by FDA.[136]

FDAMA limited the use of some postmarket controls (device tracking and postmarket surveillance) to Class II and Class III devices, eased reporting requirements of adverse events for device user facilities, eliminated mandatory reporting of adverse events by medical device distributors, and directed FDA to establish a sentinel reporting system to collect information on deaths and serious injuries or illnesses associated with the use of a medical device.[137]

User Fee Acts and the FDA Amendments Act of 2007

The *Medical Device User Fee and Modernization Act of 2002* (MDUFMA; P.L. 107-250) established a user fee program for premarket reviews of 510(k) submissions and PMA applications; user fees may not be used for other FDA or CDRH activities. MDUFMA also made targeted changes that would reduce regulatory burdens and agency workload, such as allowing establishment inspections to be conducted by accredited persons (third parties). MDUFMA was amended and clarified by two laws: *the Medical Device Technical Corrections Act of 2004* (MDTCA, P.L. 108-214), and the *Medical Device User Fee Stabilization Act of 2005* (MDUFSA, P.L. 109-43), and had its user fee provisions reauthorized by the *Medical Device User Fee Act of 2007* (MDUFA; Title II of FDAAA, see below).

The *Food and Drug Administration Amendments Act of 2007* (FDAAA; P.L. 110-85) amended the FFDCA and the Public Health Service Act to reauthorize several expiring programs (including the medical device user fee act) and to make agency-wide changes, several of which have implications for the regulation of medical devices.[138] FDAAA created incentives as well as reporting and safety requirements for manufacturers of medical devices for children; required that certain clinical trials for medical devices and some other products be publicly registered and have their results posted;[139] created requirements to reduce conflicts of interest in advisory committees for medical devices and other products;[140] and made certain other amendments to the regulation of devices.

APPENDIX B. ACRONYMS USED IN THIS REPORT

BIMO	Bioresearch Monitoring
CBER	Center for Biologics Evaluation and Research
CDRH	Center for Devices and Radiological Health
CFR	Code of Federal Regulations
CSOs	Consumer safety officers
FDA	Food and Drug Administration
FDAAA	Food and Drug Administration Amendments Act of 2007
FDAMA	Food and Drug Administration Modernization Act of 1997
FFDCA	Federal Food, Drug and Cosmetic Act
GAO	General Accountability Office
GGP	Good Guidance Practices
GHTF	Global Harmonization Task Force
GMP	Good manufacturing practices
HHS	Health and Human Services
IDE	Investigational Device Exemption
IOM	Institute of Medicine
IRB	Institutional review board
IVD	In Vitro Diagnostic
MDA	Medical Device Amendments of 1976
MDR	Medical Device Reporting
MDTCA	Medical Device Technical Corrections Act of 2004
MDUFA	Medical Device User Fee Act of 2007
MDUFMA	Medical Device User Fee and Modernization Act of 2002
MDUFSA	Medical Device User Fee Stabilization Act of 2005
NSE	Not substantially equivalent
OC	Office of Compliance
ORA	Office of Regulatory Affairs
PMA	Premarket Approval
QSR	Quality Systems Regulation
SMDA	Safe Medical Devices Act of 1990
UDI	Unique device identification

End Notes

[1] The Lewin Group, for AdvaMed, *State Economic Impact of the Medical Technology Industry,* June 7, 2010, p. 19.

[2] Jurisdiction of the centers' medical device review is governed by the FDA Intercenter Agreement between CBER and CDRH (October 31, 1991). FDA, *Devices Regulated by the Center for Biologics Evaluation and Research*, http://www.fda.gov/BiologicsBlood Vaccines/DevelopmentApprovalProcess/510kProcess/ucm133429.htm.

[3] For more information on FDA's budget, see CRS Report R41737, *Public Health Service (PHS) Agencies: Overview and Funding, FY2010-FY2012*, coordinated by C. Stephen Redhead and Pamela W. Smith; and, CRS Report RL34334, *The Food and Drug Administration: Budget and Statutory History, FY1980-FY2007*, coordinated by Judith A. Johnson.

[4] FDA also funds some device and radiological health activities with fees collected under the Mammography Quality Standards Act (MQSA, P.L. 102-539), and device user fees fund some non–device-specific activities at FDA.

[5] Price WaterhouseCoopers / National Venture Capital Association, "Medical Devices and Equipment," *Money Tree Report*, data provided by Thomson Reuters, at http://www. pwcmoneytree.com.

[6] Ernst and Young. 2010. *Pulse of the industry: Medical technology report*, p. 15.

[7] Ibid., p. 87.

[8] PwC (PricewaterhouseCoopers), *Medical Technology Innovation Scorecard: The race for global leadership*, January 2011, p. 8, http://www.pwc.com/us/en/health-industries/health-research-institute/innovation-scorecard.

[9] For example, see Barry Meier and Janet Roberts, "Hip implant complaints surge, even as the dangers are studied," *The New York Times*, August 22, 2011, pp. A1, A16; Information on recalls is available by searching the database at FDA, *Medical & Radiation Emitting Device Recalls*, http://www.accessdata.fda.gov/scripts/cdrh/cfdocs/cfRES/res.cfm.

[10] FDA, CDRH Reports, OCD FY2006: FDA Goal 3-Improving Product Quality, Safety, and Availability Through Better Manufacturing and Product Oversight, at http://www.fda.gov/ AboutFDA/CentersOffices/CDRH/CDRHReports/ucm129324.htm; and Statement of Diana Zuckerman, PhD, President of the National Research Center for Women & Families at the House of Representatives Briefing on Medical Devices, May 17, 2011, at http://www. center4research.org/2011/05/statement-of-diana-zuckerman-phd-president-of-the-national-research-center-for-women-families-at-a-house-of-representatives-briefing-on-medical-devices/.

[11] U.S. Government Accountability Office, *Medical Devices: FDA should take steps to ensure that high-risk device types are approved through the most stringent premarket review process*, GAO-09-190, January 2009; Daniel R. Levinson, *Adverse Event Reporting for Medical Devices*, Department of Health and Human Services, Office of Inspector General, Washington, DC, October 2009; and, IOM (Institute of Medicine), *Medical Devices and the Public's Health: The FDA 510(k) Clearance Process at 35 Years*, Washington, DC, July 2011.

[12] GAO regularly reports on government operations that it identifies as high risk due to their greater vulnerability to fraud, waste, abuse, mismanagement or the need for transformation to address economy, efficiency or effectiveness challenges. See GAO, *High-Risk Series: An Update*, GAO-09-271, January 2009; and GAO, *High-Risk Series: An Update*, GAO-11-278, February 2011.

[13] (21 CFR 862-892).

[14] The term *manufacturer* is used throughout this report for simplicity, but regulations also apply to any person, organization, or sponsor that submits an application to FDA to market a device.

[15] *In vitro* diagnostic products (IVDs, or laboratory tests) have their own unique premarket requirements and are not discussed further in this report.

[16] This is somewhat similar to the process FDA uses to approve a new prescription drug. For more information, see CRS Report R41983, *How FDA Approves Drugs and Regulates Their Safety and Effectiveness*, by Susan Thaul.

[17] To be a predicate, a device must have either been on the market before 1976 when the Medical Device Amendments (MDA) took effect, or it could have been cleared for marketing after 1976, but must have the same intended use as a device classified in the Code of Federal Regulations (CFR).

[18] U.S. Government Accountability Office, *Medical Devices: FDA should take steps to ensure that high-risk device types are approved through the most stringent premarket review process*, GAO-09-190, January 2009, p. 9.

[19] FFDCA §513(a)(1); see also 21 CFR §860.3(c). As of 2009, the agency has classified over 1,700 distinct types of devices. The device types are organized in the Code of Federal Regulations (CFR) in 16 *classification panels*, such as "cardiovascular devices" or "ear, nose, and throat devices." FDA, *Device Classification*, June 18, 2009, http://www.fda.gov/MedicalDevices/DeviceRegulationandGuidance/Overview/ClassifyYourDevice/default.htm.

[20] See FDA, *General and Special Controls*, April 30, 2009, http://www.fda.gov/MedicalDevices/DeviceRegulationandGuidance/Overview/GeneralandSpecialControls/default.htm.

[21] 21 CFR 807.20

[22] 21 CFR 820

[23] 21 CFR 801 or 809.10.

[24] FFDCA §513(a)(1)(A).

[25] See 21 CFR 862 to 892.

[26] FFDCA §513(a)(1)(B).

[27] IOM, *Medical Devices and the Public's Health: The FDA 510(k) Clearance Process at 35 Years*, Washington, DC, July 2011, p. 40.

[28] FDA, Overview of Medical Device Regulation, Medical Device Classification, Class I/II Exemptions, at http://www.fda.gov/MedicalDevices/DeviceRegulationandGuidance/Overview/ClassifyYourDevice/ucm051549.htm.

[29] FFDCA §513(a)(1)(C).

[30] FFDCA §513(f)(2).

[31] IOM, *Medical Devices and the Public's Health: The FDA 510(k) Clearance Process at 35 Years*, Washington, DC, July 2011, p. 81.

[32] FDA, Overview of Medical Device Regulation, General and Special Controls, at http://www.fda.gov/MedicalDevices/DeviceRegulationandGuidance/Overview/GeneralandSpecialControls/default.htm.

[33] FDA, CDRH Transparency, 515 Program Initiative, at http://www.fda.gov/AboutFDA/CentersOffices/CDRH/CDRHTransparency/ucm240310.htm.

[34] Diana M. Zuckerman, Paul Brown, and Steven Nissen, "Medical device recalls and the FDA approval process," *Archives of Internal Medicine*, Online publication 2011, p. E2.

[35] Ibid., p. E2.

[36] FDA, CDRH Transparency, 515 Program Status, at http://www.fda.gov/AboutFDA/CentersOffices/CDRH/CDRHTransparency/ucm240318.htm.

[37] FDA, CDRH Transparency, 515 Program Initiative, at http://www.fda.gov/AboutFDA/CentersOffices/CDRH/CDRHTransparency/ucm240310.htm.

[38] U.S. Congress, Senate Special Committee on Aging, *A Delicate Balance: FDA and the Reform of the Medical Device Approval Process*, Testimony of William Maisel, Deputy Center Director for Science, FDA/CDRH, 112th Cong., 1st sess., April 13, 2011.

[39] For guidance on the procedures established, see *Early Collaboration Meetings Under the FDA Modernization Act*; Final Guidance for Industry and CDRH Staff, February 28, 2001, at

http://www.fda.gov/MedicalDevices/DeviceRegulationandGuidance/GuidanceDocuments/ucm073604.htm.

[40] U.S. Congress, Senate Committee on Health, Education, Labor, and Pensions, *Medical Devices: Protecting Patients and Promoting Innovation*, 112th Cong., 1st sess., November 15, 2011.

[41] A device is adulterated if it includes any filthy, putrid, or decomposed substance, or if it is prepared, packed, or held under unsanitary conditions. The FFDCA further states that a device is adulterated if its container contains any poisonous or deleterious substance, or if its strength, purity or quality varies significantly from what the manufacturer claims. For higher class devices, a device can be considered adulterated if it fails to meet performance requirements outlined in its approval, or if it is in violation of other Good Manufacturing Practice requirements.

[42] A device is misbranded when all or part of the labeling (i.e., the FDA-approved printed material providing information about the device) is false, misleading, or missing.

[43] FDA, "Medical Device User Fee Rates for Fiscal Year 2010," 74 *Federal Register* 38444-38449, August 3, 2009;http://edocket.access.gpo.gov/2009/E9-18456.htm.

[44] U.S. Government Accountability Office, *Medical Devices: FDA should take steps to ensure that high-risk device types are approved through the most stringent premarket review process*, GAO-09-190, January 2009.

[45] U.S. Congress, Senate Committee on Health, Education, Labor, and Pensions, *Medical Devices: Protecting Patients and Promoting Innovation*, Testimony of Jeffrey Shuren, Director CDRH, FDA, 112th Cong., 1st sess., November 15, 2011, http://help.senate.gov/imo/media/doc/Shuren.pdf.

[46] IOM, *Public Health Effectiveness of the FDA 510(k) Clearance Process: Measuring Postmarket Performance and Other Select Topics*, Workshop Report, Washington, DC, 2011, pp. 12 and 78.

[47] U.S. Government Accountability Office, *Medical Devices: FDA should take steps to ensure that high-risk device types are approved through the most stringent premarket review process*, GAO-09-190, January 2009, p. 18.

[48] Ibid., p. 27.

[49] FDA, Medical Devices, 510(k) Submission Methods, at http://www.fda.gov/MedicalDevices/DeviceRegulationandGuidance/HowtoMarketYourDevice/PremarketSubmissions/PremarketNotification510k/ ucm134034.htm

[50] IOM, *Public Health Effectiveness of the FDA 510(k) Clearance Process: Measuring Postmarket Performance and Other Select Topics*, Workshop Report, Washington, DC, 2011, pp. 12 and 79.

[51] FDA, *How to Prepare a Traditional 510(k)*, September 14, 2009; http://www.fda.gov/MedicalDevices/DeviceRegulationandGuidance/HowtoMarketYourDevice/PremarketSubmissions/PremarketNotification510k/ucm134572.htm#link_4.

[52] Diana M. Zuckerman, Paul Brown, and Steven Nissen, "Medical device recalls and the FDA approval process," *Archives of Internal Medicine*, Online publication 2011, p. E4.

[53] 21 CFR 807.100(a).

[54] 21 CFR 807.87(l).

[55] The FDA time clock (i.e., review cycle) begins when FDA receives the 510(k) and ends with the date that FDA issues either a request for additional information or a decision. More than one cycle may occur before FDA issues its final decision.

[56] 21 CFR 10.115. FDA continually accepts public comment on any draft or final guidance document.

[57] 21 CFR 861.

[58] Design controls are a series of predetermined checks, verifications, and specifications that are built into the manufacturing process to validate the quality of the product throughout the process. These can include defining the personnel responsible for implementing steps in the development and manufacturing process, defining specifications and standards for assessing

the quality of the materials that go into making the product, designing specifications for accepting and rejecting different batches or lots of final product, and requirements for maintaining appropriate records.

[59] 21 CFR 820.30.

[60] FDA, *New Section 513(f)(2)—Evaluation of Automatic Class III Designation, Guidance for Industry and CDRH Staff*, February 19, 1998, http://www.fda.gov/MedicalDevices/DeviceRegulationandGuidance/GuidanceDocuments/ucm080195.htm.

[61] Food and Drug Administration, "FDA Seeks Comment on Streamlined Review of Lower Risk, New Technology, Devices," press release, September 30, 2011, http://www.fda.gov/NewsEvents/Newsroom/PressAnnouncements/ucm274008.htm.

[62] 21 CFR 814.

[63] PMAs can also use studies from the medical literature (a "paper PMA").

[64] See 21 CFR 812. Devices are exempt from IDE requirements when testing is noninvasive, does not require invasive sampling, does not introduce energy into a subject, and is not stand alone (i.e., is not used for diagnosis without confirmation by other methods or medically established procedures). See 21 CFR 812.2(c)(3).

[65] FDA, *Device Advice: Investigational Device Exemption (IDE)*, July 9, 2009, http://www.fda.gov/MedicalDevices/DeviceRegulationandGuidance/HowtoMarketYourDevice/InvestigationalDeviceExemptionIDE/default.htm.

[66] FDA, "FDA seeks comment on proposed guidance for high-quality clinical studies," FDA, press release, August 15, 2011, http://www.fda.gov/NewsEvents/Newsroom/PressAnnouncements/ucm268000.htm; and, "FDA issues two draft guidance documents to facilitate investigational medical device studies in humans," press release, November 10, 2011, http://www.fda.gov/NewsEvents/Newsroom/PressAnnouncements/ucm279459.htm.

[67] An IRB is a group, generally comprised volunteers, that examines proposed and ongoing scientific research to ensure that human subjects are properly protected. For further information, see CRS Report RL32909, *Federal Protection for Human Research Subjects: An Analysis of the Common Rule and Its Interactions with FDA Regulations and the HIPAA Privacy Rule*, by Erin D. Williams.

[68] 21 CFR 820.

[69] For further information, see CRS Report RS22691, *FDA Advisory Committee Conflict of Interest*, by Erin D. Williams.

[70] 21 CFR 14.

[71] FDA, *FY2010 Performance Report to the Congress for the Medical Device User Fee Amendments of 2007*, http://www.fda.gov/downloads/AboutFDA/ReportsManualsForms/Reports/UserFeeReports/PerformanceReports/MDUFMA/UCM243386.pdf. See also 21 CFR 814.40.

[72] FDA officials meet with industry leaders to agree upon mutually acceptable fee types, amounts, exceptions, and performance goals. The agreement specifies that, in return for the additional resources provided by medical device user fees, FDA is expected to meet performance goals defined in a letter, generally referred to as the "FDA Commitment Letter," from the HHS Secretary to the Chairmen and Ranking Minority Members of the Committee on Health, Education, Labor and Pensions of the U.S. Senate and the Committee on Energy and Commerce of the U.S. House of Representatives. This process is similar to the one used for prescription drug user fees under the Prescription Drug User Fee Act (PDUFA). For further information on PDUFA, see CRS Report RL33914, *The Prescription Drug User Fee Act: History Through the 2007 PDUFA IV Reauthorization*, by Susan Thaul.

[73] FFDCA §201(k)

[74] FFDCA §201(m)

[75] United States v. Research Laboratories, Inc., 126 F.2d 42 (9th Cir. 1942).

[76] 21 CFR 801

[77] 21 CFR 801.405 to 801.437. Denture repair kits, impact resistant lenses in sunglasses and eyeglasses, ozone emission levels, chlorofluorocarbon propellants, hearing aids, menstrual tampons, chlorofluorocarbons or other ozone depleting substances, latex condoms, and devices containing natural rubber.

[78] 21 CFR 820.120

[79] FFDCA §520; 21 CFR 820

[80] FDA, *Medical Devices: 1. The Quality System Regulation*, June 18, 2009, http://www.fda.gov/MedicalDevices/DeviceRegulationandGuidance/PostmarketRequirements/QualitySystemsRegulations/MedicalDeviceQualitySystemsManual/ucm122391.htm.

[81] IOM, *Medical Devices and the Public's Health: The FDA 510(k) Clearance Process at 35 Years*, Washington, DC, July 2011, p. 99.

[82] FFDCA §522.

[83] 21 USC 355 note

[84] FFDCA §519(a)

[85] The searchable MDR database for devices is publically accessible at http://www.accessdata.fda.gov/scripts/cdrh/ cfdocs/cfmdr/search.CFM.

[86] 21 CFR 803.10(c)(1) and 803.10(c)(2)

[87] 21 CFR 803.10(a)(1)(i).

[88] 21 CFR 803.10(a)(1)(ii).

[89] 21 CFR 803.10(a)(2) and 803.33.

[90] FDA, "Proposed Rule, Medical Device Reporting: Electronic Submission Requirements," 74 *Federal Register*42203-42217, August 21, 2009; and FDA, "Draft Guidance for Industry, User Facilities, and Food and Drug Administration Staff; eMDR—Electronic Medical Device Reporting; Availability," 74 *Federal Register* Page 42310, August 21, 2009.

[91] Daniel R. Levinson, *Adverse Event Reporting for Medical Devices*, HHS Office of Inspector General, OEI-01-08-00110, October 2009, http://oig.hhs.gov/oei/reports/oei-01-08-00110.pdf.

[92] FDA, *Medical Device Tracking*, May 13, 2009, http://www.fda.gov/MedicalDevices/DeviceRegulationandGuidance/PostmarketRequirements/MedicalDeviceTracking/default.htm#link_2.

[93] 21 CFR 821

[94] A device user facility means a hospital, ambulatory surgical facility, nursing home, or outpatient treatment facility which is not a physician's office. A current list of the devices for which tracking is required can be found at http://www.fda.gov/MedicalDevices/DeviceRegulationandGuidance/PostmarketRequirements/MedicalDeviceTracking/default.htm#link_2.

[95] FFDCA §505(k); 21 USC 355

[96] FFDCA §1003(b)(2)(c)

[97] U.S. Food and Drug Administration, *The Sentinel Initiative: Access to Electronic Healthcare Data for More Than 25 Million Lives*, July 2010, http://www.fda.gov/downloads/Safety/FDAsSentinelInitiative/UCM233360.pdf.

[98] Rachel E. Behrman, Joshua S. Benner, and Jeffrey S. Brown, et al., "Developing the Sentinel System—A National Resource for Evidence Development," *The New England Journal of Medicine*, vol. 364, no. 6 (February 10, 2011), pp.498-499. The Sentinel Initiative is focused on electronic claims data held by health plans. Importantly, the plans retain control over the patient-level data within their own data firewalls and provide only aggregated information to FDA.

[99] IOM, *Medical Devices and the Public's Health: The FDA 510(k) Clearance Process at 35 Years*, Washington, DC, July 2011, p. 106.

[100] Information on the current status of the Sentinel Initiative is available at http://www.fda.gov/Safety/FDAsSentinelInitiative/default.htm.

[101] FFDCA §519(f); 21 USC 360i

[102] FDA, "Unique Device Identification for Postmarket Surveillance and Enforcement; Public Workshop," 76 *Federal Register* 43691-43693, July 21, 2011.

[103] FDA, Center for Devices and Radiological Health, *CDRH FY 2010 Strategic Priorities*, p. 6, http://www.fda.gov/downloads/AboutFDA/CentersOffices/CDRH/CDRHVisionandMission/UCM197648.pdf.

[104] Alaina Bush, "CER, Safety uses eyed as part of FDA device identification rule," *Inside Health Reform*, vol. 3, no. 39 (September 22, 2011).

[105] Meeting information, reports and current status of the UDI system can be found at http://www.fda.gov/MedicalDevices/DeviceRegulationandGuidance/UniqueDeviceIdentification/default.htm

[106] GHTF website is at http://www.ghtf.org/.

[107] GHTF SC UDI Ad Hoc Working Group, *Unique Device Identification (UDI) System for Medical Devices*, Global Harmonization Task Force, GHTF/AHWG-UDI/N2R3:2011, September 16, 2011, http://www.ghtf.org/documents/ ahwg/AHWG-UDI-N2R3.pdf.

[108] See ORA at http://www.fda.gov/AboutFDA/CentersOffices/ORA/default.htm.

[109] Warning letters are publically available on FDA's website at http://www.fda.gov/ICECI/EnforcementActions/WarningLetters/default.htm.

[110] Recall does not include market withdrawal or a stock recovery. A market withdrawal is a firm's removal or correction of a distributed product for a minor violation that does not violate the law and would not be subject to legal action by FDA (e.g., normal stock rotation practices, routine equipment adjustments and repairs, etc.). Stock recovery involves correction of a problem before product is shipped (i.e., is still in the manufacturer's control).

[111] 21 CFR 7

[112] 21 CFR 806.

[113] 21 CFR 810. See out-of-print CRS Report RL34167, *The FDA's Authority to Recall Products*, by Vanessa K. Burrows (available from the author upon request).

[114] The main page for recalls, market withdrawals, and safety alerts for all FDA-regulated products ishttp://www.fda.gov/opacom/7alerts.html.

[115] U.S. Congress, House Committee on Interstate and Foreign Commerce, *Medical Device Amendments of 1976*, to accompany H.R. 11124, 94th Cong., 2nd sess., February 29, 1976, H. Rept. 94-853, p. 6.

[116] Ibid. "A device is adulterated if it includes any filthy, putrid, or decomposed substance, or if it is prepared, packed, or held under unsanitary conditions. A device is misbranded if its labeling is false or misleading; unless it identifies the manufacturer, packer, or distributor and quantity of contents; if required labeling statements are not conspicuous; if it fails to bear adequate directions for use or adequate warnings; or if it is dangerous to health when used as indicated."

[117] Ibid.

[118] Ibid., p. 7.

[119] Ibid., p. 7-8.

[120] Ibid., p. 8. By 1975, the Dalkon Shield had been linked to at least 16 deaths and 25 miscarriages, numerous cases of pelvic perforation and pelvic infection, removal of the IUD for medical reasons, and pregnancies due to IUD failure. As of February 1976, more than 500 lawsuits seeking compensatory and punitive damages totaling more than $400 million were pending against the manufacturer of the Dalkon Shield. IOM, *Medical Devices and the Public's Health: The FDA 510(k) Clearance Process at 35 Years*, Washington, DC, July 2011, p. 172, http://www.iom.edu/Reports/2011/Medical-Devices-and-the-Publics-Health-The-FDA-510k-Clearance-Process-at-35-Years.aspx.

[121] U.S. Congress, House Committee on Interstate and Foreign Commerce, *Medical Device Amendments of 1976*, to accompany H.R. 11124, 94th Cong., 2nd sess., February 29, 1976, H. Rept. 94-853, p. 8-9.

[122] An instrument, apparatus, implement, machine, contrivance, implant, in vitro reagent, or other similar or related article, including any component, part, or accessory, which is (1)

recognized in the official National Formulary, or the United States Pharmacopeia, or any supplement to them; (2) intended for use in the diagnosis of disease or other conditions, or in the cure, mitigation, treatment, or prevention of disease, in man or other animals; or (3) intended to affect the structure or any function of the body of man or other animals, and which does not achieve any of its principal intended purposes through chemical action within or on the body of man or other animals and which is not dependent upon being metabolized for the achievement of its primary intended purposes. The definition was changed in 1992 from "any of its principal intended purposes" to "its primary intended purposes." Current definition at FFDCA §201(h), (21 U.S.C. 321).

[123] The law has since been amended to exempt many (Class I) products from some general controls or to limit the application of general controls to subsets of (Class II or Class III) products that pose higher risks. IOM, *Medical Devices and the Public's Health: The FDA 510(k) Clearance Process at 35 Years*, Washington, DC, July 2011, p. 175.

[124] Preamendment devices were presumed to be marketable. They did not undergo premarket review and could be legally marketed unless FDA required their removal. After classifying the preamendment devices, FDA used them as the first cadre of "predicate" devices in order to demonstrate substantial equivalence.

[125] Ibid., p. 24.

[126] Ibid., p. 177.

[127] Ibid., p. 25.

[128] Ibid., p. 179.

[129] Ibid. p. 180.

[130] FFDCA §515(i).

[131] IOM, *Medical Devices and the Public's Health: The FDA 510(k) Clearance Process at 35 Years*, Washington, DC, July 2011, p. 205.

[132] FFDCA §513(i).

[133] IOM, *Medical Devices and the Public's Health: The FDA 510(k) Clearance Process at 35 Years*, Washington, DC, July 2011, p. 28.

[134] Ibid., p. 213.

[135] FFDCA §513(i)(1)(D).

[136] FFDCA §515(d)(5).

[137] FFDCA §519 and §522. A device user facility means a hospital, ambulatory surgical facility, nursing home, or outpatient treatment facility which is not a physician's office.

[138] See CRS Report RL34465, *FDA Amendments Act of 2007 (P.L. 110-85)*, by Erin D. Williams and Susan Thaul.

[139] See the Clinical Trials Databases section of CRS Report RL34465, *FDA Amendments Act of 2007 (P.L. 110-85)*, by Erin D. Williams and Susan Thaul.

[140] FDA uses advisory committees to gain independent advice from outside experts. See CRS Report RS22691, *FDA Advisory Committee Conflict of Interest*, by Erin D. Williams.

In: Medical Devices and the FDA ISBN: 978-1-62257-674-6
Editors: Gil Frazier and Brady Malone © 2013 Nova Science Publishers, Inc.

Chapter 2

THE FDA MEDICAL DEVICE USER FEE PROGRAM*

Judith A. Johnson

On June 20, 2012, the House of Representatives passed, by voice vote and under suspension of the rules, S. 3187 (EAH), the Food and Drug Administration Safety and Innovation Act, as amended. This bill would reauthorize the FDA prescription drug and medical device user fee programs (which would otherwise expire on September 30, 2012), create new user fee programs for generic and biosimilar drug approvals, and make other revisions to other FDA drug and device approval processes. It reflects bicameral compromise on earlier versions of the bill (S. 3187 [ES], which passed the Senate on May 24, 2012, and H.R. 5651 [EH], which passed the House on May 30, 2012).

SUMMARY

The Food and Drug Administration (FDA) is the agency responsible for the regulation of medical devices. These are a wide range of products that are used to diagnose, treat, monitor, or prevent a disease or condition in a patient. A company must obtain FDA's prior approval or clearance before marketing

* This is an edited, reformatted and augmented version of the Congressional Research Service Publication, CRS Report for Congress R42508, dated June 25, 2012.

many medical devices in the United States. The Center for Devices and Radiological Health (CDRH) within FDA is primarily responsible for medical device review and regulation.

Congress first gave FDA the authority to collect user fees from medical device companies in the Medical Device User Fee and Modernization Act of 2002 (P.L. 107-250). The purpose of the user fee program is to help reduce the time in which FDA can review and make decisions on marketing applications. Lengthy review times affect the industry, which waits to market its products, and patients, who wait to use these products. The user fee law provides a revenue stream for FDA; in conjunction, the agency negotiates with industry to set *performance goals* for the premarket review of medical devices. Reauthorization of FDA's medical device user fees last occurred in 2007, just before the FDA's authority would expire, via the Medical Device User Fee Amendments of 2007 (MDUFA II). Current authority will expire on October 1, 2012.

On February 1, 2012, FDA announced that it had reached "an agreement in principle" with the medical device industry on proposed recommendations for the second reauthorization—referred to as MDUFA III. A draft MDUFA III package, composed of statutory language and the FDA-industry agreement on performance goals and procedures, was posted on the FDA website on March 14, 2012, and a public meeting describing the draft was held on March 28, 2012. The 30-day comment period on the draft ended April 16, 2012. Following review of the comments, FDA may revise the recommendation and then is to submit the final package to Congress.

Since medical device user fees were first collected in FY2003, they have comprised an increasing proportion of FDA's device budget. Medical device user fees have raised a number of concerns, prompting Congress to carefully consider issues such as which agency activities could use fees, how user fees can be kept from supplanting federal funding, and which companies should qualify as a small business and pay a reduced fee.

Congress is also considering reauthorization of the Prescription Drug User Fee Act (PDUFA) as well as new proposals for a Generic Drug User Fee Act and a Biosimilars User Fee Act. It is likely that these three will be combined with MDUFA III along with a variety of related and unrelated issues. Because of the importance of user fees to FDA's budget, PDUFA and MDUFA are considered to be "must pass" legislation, and Congress has often in the past included language to address a range of other concerns. For example, MDUFA II included provisions about the extent to which FDA can delegate activities to third parties, a unique device identification system, and reporting requirements for devices linked to serious injuries or deaths. House and Senate committees are circulating discussion drafts that contain many proposals that would affect medical device regulation. FDA has indicated that some of these pending reforms could conflict with what was negotiated with industry in the MDUFA III proposal. Some reforms are of concern because they would require more agency resources; others were discussed during the user fee negotiations and were set aside. If MDUFA reauthorization does not occur by early summer, federal regulations require that reduction-in-force notices be sent out in July 2012, giving 60 days' advance notice to about 250 FDA employees that their employment under the MDUFA program would end September 30, 2012.

INTRODUCTION

In 2002, the Medical Device User Fee and Modernization Act (MDUFMA) gave the Food and Drug Administration (FDA) the authority to collect fees from the medical device industry.[1] User fees and direct appropriations from Congress fund review of medical devices by the FDA. Medical devices are a wide range of products that are used to diagnose, treat, monitor, or prevent a disease or condition in a patient. The Federal Food, Drug and Cosmetic Act (FFDCA) defines a medical device as

> an instrument, apparatus, implement, machine, contrivance, implant, in vitro reagent, or other similar or related article, including any component, part, or accessory, which is (1) recognized in the official National Formulary, or the United States Pharmacopeia, or any supplement to them, (2) intended for use in the diagnosis of disease or other conditions, or in the cure, mitigation, treatment, or prevention of disease, in man or other animals, or (3) intended to affect the structure or any function of the body of man or other animals, and which does not achieve its primary intended purposes through chemical action within or on the body of man or other animals and which is not dependent upon being metabolized for the achievement of its primary intended purposes. (FFDCA §201(h), 21 U.S.C. 301 §201(h))

According to FDA, examples of medical devices "range from simple tongue depressors and bedpans to complex programmable pacemakers with micro-chip technology and laser surgical devices."[2] Medical devices also include in vitro diagnostic products, reagents, test kits, and certain electronic radiation-emitting products with medical applications, such as diagnostic ultrasound products, x-ray machines, and medical lasers.

Manufacturers must obtain FDA approval or clearance before marketing many medical devices in the United States. The Center for Devices and Radiological Health (CDRH) has primary responsibility within FDA for medical device premarket review.[3] The purpose of user fees is to support the FDA's medical device premarket review program and to help reduce the time it takes the agency to review and make decisions on marketing applications. Prior to 2002, multiple government reports, as early as 1983, indicated that FDA had insufficient resources for its medical devices premarket review program.[4] Lengthy review times affect the industry, which waits to market its products, and patients, who wait to use these products. The user fee law provides revenue for FDA; in conjunction, the agency negotiates with industry to set *performance goals* for the premarket review of medical devices. The medical device user fee program was modeled after the Prescription Drug User Fee Act (PDUFA).[5]

Like the prescription drug and animal drug user fee programs, the medical device user fee program has been authorized in five-year increments.[6] FDA's medical device user fee authorities were reauthorized just before their expiration by the Medical Device User Fee Amendments of 2007 (MDUFA).[7] The agency's current authority to collect medical device user fees will expire on October 1, 2012.

On February 1, 2012, FDA announced that it had reached "an agreement in principle" with the medical device industry on proposed recommendations for the reauthorization of the medical device user fee program.[8] Referred to as MDUFA III, a draft of the negotiated package— composed of statutory language and the FDA-industry agreement on performance goals and procedures—was posted on the FDA website on March 14, 2012.[9] A public meeting describing the draft was held on March 28, 2012. The 30-day comment period on the draft ended April 16, 2012. Following review of the comments, FDA may revise the recommendation and then is to submit the final package to Congress.

This report describes current law regarding medical device user fees, the impact of MDUFA on FDA review time of various medical device applications and the agency's medical device program budget, the MDUFA III proposal (legislative language and performance goals agreement), and issues that Congress is likely to take up as it works on the reauthorization of the medical device user fee program. **Appendix E** provides a list of acronyms used in this report.

CURRENT LAW

The Medical Device Amendments of 1976 (P.L. 94-295) was the first major legislation passed to address the premarket review of medical devices. User fees to support the FDA's medical device premarket review program were first authorized by Congress in 2002, 10 years after Congress had provided the authority for prescription drug user fees via PDUFA. For prescription drugs, the manufacturer must pay a fee for each new drug application (NDA) that is submitted to FDA for premarket review. In contrast, most medical devices are exempt from premarket review and do not pay a user fee. Premarket review and payment of the associated fee is required for about a third of the medical devices listed with FDA (see **Figure 1**).

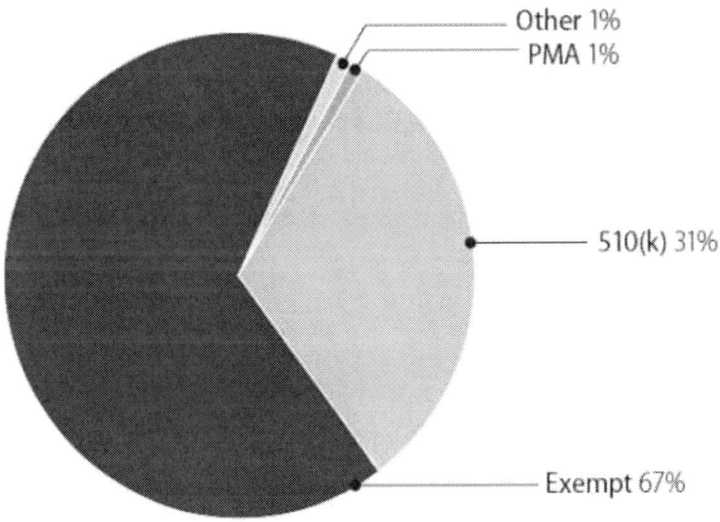

Source: Government Accountability Office, January 2009, GAO-09-190, p. 9.

Notes: "Other" includes devices that were allowed to enter the market via other means, such as through the humanitarian device exemption process that allows market entry, without adherence to certain requirements, for devices benefiting patients with rare diseases or conditions. See "Exemptions and Discounted Fees." Non-exempt devices are reviewed by FDA via the PMA (premarket approval) process or the 510(k) notification. See "FDA Premarket Review of Medical Devices."

Figure 1. Medical Devices Listed with FDA, FY2003-FY2007, by Premarket Review Process.

FDA Premarket Review of Medical Devices

FDA classifies devices based on the risk to the patient: low-risk devices are Class I, medium-risk are Class II, and high-risk are Class III. Low-risk medical devices (Class I) and a very small number of moderate-risk (Class II) medical devices are exempt from premarket review. In general, for moderate-risk and high-risk medical devices, there are two pathways that manufacturers can use to bring such devices to market with FDA's permission.[10]

One pathway consists of conducting clinical studies, then submitting a premarket approval (PMA) application with evidence providing reasonable assurance that the device is safe and effective. The PMA process is generally used for novel and high-risk devices and is typically lengthy and expensive. It results in a type of FDA permission called *approval.*

Another pathway involves submitting a premarket notification submission—also known as a 510(k), after the section in the FFDCA that authorized this type of notification. With the 510(k), the manufacturer demonstrates that the device is substantially equivalent to a device already on the market (a predicate device) that does not require a PMA. The 510(k) process is unique to medical devices and results in FDA clearance. Substantial equivalence is determined by comparing the performance characteristics of a new device with those of a predicate device.

Medical Device User Fees

Premarket review by FDA—both PMA and 510(k)—requires the payment of a user fee. FDA typically *evaluates* more than 4,000 510(k) notifications and about 40 original PMA applications each year.[11] Since MDUFA II reauthorization in 2007, FDA *cleared* over 13,000 510(k) devices and *approved* 106 PMAs.[12] According to CDRH Director Jeffrey Shuren, for FY2010, user fees collected under MDUFA "fund only about 20% of the device review program"; in contrast, user fees collected under the PDUFA account for over 60% of the drug review program's budget.[13]

There are also fees for when a manufacturer requests approval of a significant change in the design or performance of a device approved via the PMA pathway.[14] This is called a Panel-Track Supplement when it is necessary for FDA to evaluate significant clinical data in order to make a decision on approval of the supplement. If a manufacturer requests approval of a change in aspects of an approved device, such as its design, specifications, or labeling, this is called a 180-Day PMA Supplement. In this case, FDA either does not require new clinical data or requires only limited clinical data. When a manufacturer requests approval for a minor change to an approved device, such as a minor change in the design or labeling, this is called a Real-Time PMA Supplement. With a Premarket Report, a manufacturer requests the approval of a high-risk device, originally approved for single use (one patient, one procedure), for reprocessing to allow additional use.

The original 2002 user fee law had only authorized FDA to collect fees for premarket review, such as for PMA applications or 510(k) notifications. The 2007 reauthorization—MDUFA II— added two new types of annual fees in order to generate a more stable revenue stream for the agency. According to FDA, there were fluctuations in the numbers submitted from year to year, and fee revenues repeatedly fell short of expectations.[15] MDUFA II added *establishment fees*, paid annually by most device establishments registered with FDA, and *product fees*, paid annually for high-risk (Class III) devices for which periodic reporting is required.

The annual fees were projected to generate about 50% of the total device fee revenue from FY2008 to FY2012.[16] MDUFA II also added two new application fees, the 30-Day Notice and 513(g) application, and substantially lowered all the existing application fee amounts (see **Table C-1**). A manufacturer uses a 30-Day Notice when requesting to make modifications to manufacturing procedures or methods of manufacture affecting the safety and effectiveness of the device, and a manufacturer requests information on the classification of a device with a 513(g) application.[17]

Other than the establishment fee, the amount of each type of user fee is set as a percentage of the PMA fee, also called the *base fee*. The law prescribes both the base fee amount for each fiscal year, and the percentage of the base fee that constitutes most other fees. For example, the 510(k) fee is equal to 1.84% of the PMA fee. MDUFA II raised the PMA fee by 8.5% per year from FY2008 to FY2012[18] (see **Table C-1**).

FDA asserted that this annual increase would ensure that fee revenues contribute their expected share to total program costs, and would provide industry with stability and predictability in the fee revenues it would expect to pay.[19] The amount of the establishment fee (also known as the *establishment registration fee*) was authorized under MDUFA II to rise 8.5% per year from FY2008 to FY2012[20] (see **Table C-1**).

Exemptions and Discounted Fees

Certain types of medical devices, sponsors of medical device PMA applications or 510(k) notifications, and medical device manufacturers are exempt from paying fees, and small businesses pay a reduced rate.[21] Humanitarian Device Exemption (HDE) applications are exempt from user fees, other than establishment fees.[22] An HDE exempts devices that meet certain criteria from the effectiveness requirements of premarket approval. Devices intended solely for pediatric use are exempt from fees other than establishment fees.[23] If an applicant obtains an exemption under this provision, and later submits a supplement for adult use, that supplement is subject to the fee then in effect for an original PMA.

State and federal government entities are exempt from fees for a PMA, premarket report, supplement, 510(k), and establishment registration unless the device is to be distributed commercially. Indian tribes are exempted from having to pay establishment registration fees, unless the device is to be distributed commercially. Other than an establishment fee, the FDA cannot charge a fee for premarket applications for biologics licenses and licenses for biosimilar or interchangeable products if products are licensed exclusively for further manufacturing use.[24]

Under a program authorized by Congress, FDA accredits third parties, allowing them to conduct the initial review of 510(k)s for the purpose of classification of certain devices.[25] The purpose is to improve the efficiency and timeliness of FDA's 510(k) process. No FDA fee is assessed for 510(k) submissions reviewed by accredited third parties, although the third parties charge manufacturers a fee for their services.[26]

In MDUFA II, Congress amended the process of qualifying for small business user fee discounts in response to frustrations expressed by domestic and foreign companies that had difficulties with the requirements. Small businesses—those with gross receipts below a certain amount—pay reduced user fees and have some fees waived altogether.[27] These fee reductions and exemptions are important, because many device companies are small businesses.[28]

Under current law, whether a device company is considered a small business eligible for fee reductions or waivers depends on the particular fee. Small businesses reporting under $30 million in gross receipts or sales are exempt from fees for their first PMA. Proof of receipts may consist of IRS tax documents or qualifying documentation from a foreign government. Companies with annual gross sales or receipts of $100 million or less pay at a rate of 50% of the 510(k) user fee, 30-day notice, request for classification information, and 25% of most other user fees.[29] Small businesses must pay the full amount of the establishment fees.

2007 GAO Study

A March 2007 Government Accountability Office (GAO) report analyzed company revenue information for 50% of the "4,500 device applications subject to user fees that were submitted in FY2006." The remaining 50% of applications "were likely submitted by private companies that did not qualify as small businesses," and GAO was "unable to identify the number of these companies." For the companies that GAO was able to analyze, the report found that 95% of the 697 companies qualifying as small businesses in FY2006 had revenues below $30 million. Of these 697 companies, "two-thirds submitted at least one device application subject to user fees during that year. These companies were responsible for about 20% of the approximately 4,500 device applications subject to user fees that were submitted to FDA in FY2006." GAO also analyzed the annual revenue for 258 publicly traded companies that submitted applications subject to user fees and did not qualify as small businesses in FY2006. Of these 258 companies, 155 (60%) had annual revenue higher than $500 million, 47 companies were above $100 million but at or below $500 million, and 56 companies were at or below the $100 million threshold for small business qualification. GAO did not determine why these companies were not qualified as small businesses. These 258 publicly traded companies were responsible for about 30% of the approximately 4,500 applications subject to user fees submitted to FDA in FY2006.

Source: GAO, "Food and Drug Administration: Revenue Information on Certain Companies Participating in the Medical Device User Fee Program," GAO-07-571R (March 30, 2007), at http://www.gao.gov/assets/100/94743.pdf.

Use of User Fees

A key element of FDA user fee laws—both MDUFA and PDUFA—is that the user fees are to supplement congressional appropriations, not replace them. The law includes complex formulas, called triggers, to enforce that goal. FDA may collect and use MDUFA fees only if the direct appropriations for the activities involved in the premarket review of medical devices and for FDA activities overall remain at a level at least equal (adjusted for inflation) to the pre-MDUFA budget.[30]

Other MDUFA Requirements

Over time, Congress has changed PDUFA to allow user fee revenue to be used for not only FDA activities related to premarket review but also the review of postmarket safety information associated with a drug. In contrast, MDUFA revenue can be used only for activities associated with FDA review of PMAs, 510(k)s, supplements, and reports. The law states that fees "shall only be collected and available to defray increases in the costs of resources allocated for the *process for the review of device applications*."[31]

MDUFA II added a new Section 738A regarding required reports and outlining the reauthorization process. This section required the Secretary to submit annual fiscal and performance reports for FY2008 through FY2012 to the Senate Committee on Health, Education, Labor, and Pensions, and the House Committee on Energy and Commerce. Fiscal reports address the implementation of FDA's authority to collect medical device user fees, as well as FDA's use of the fees. Performance reports address FDA's progress toward and future plans for achieving the fee-related performance goals identified in the agreement.

The new section also directed the FDA to develop a reauthorization proposal for FY2013 through FY2017 in consultation with specified congressional committees, scientific and academic experts, health care professionals, patient and consumer advocacy groups, and the regulated industry.[32] Prior to negotiations with industry, FDA was required to request public input, hold a public meeting, and publish public comments on the agency's website. During negotiations with industry, FDA was mandated to hold monthly discussions with patient and consumer advocacy groups to receive their suggestions and discuss their views on the reauthorization. After negotiations with industry were completed, FDA was required to present the recommendations to certain congressional committees, publish the recommendations in the *Federal Register*, provide a 30-day public comment period, hold another public meeting to receive views from stakeholders, and revise the recommendations as necessary. As explained earlier, the FDA missed the new statutory deadline that required the transmittal of the revised

These industry representatives noted that FDA "guidance documents are n unclear, out of date, and not comprehensive."[46] They also stated that er sponsors submit their applications to FDA, insufficient communication n FDA prevents sponsors from learning about deficiencies in their missions early in FDA's review.

According to one of these stakeholders, if FDA communicated these ciencies earlier in the process, sponsors would be able to correct them and ıld be less likely to receive a request for additional information."[47] Two ustry representatives noted that "review criteria sometimes change after a nsor submits an application," and one industry representative stated that iteria sometimes change when the FDA reviewer assigned to the mission changes during the review."[48] The February 2012 GAO report nts out that FDA has taken a number of actions to address the issues of the ustry representative.

For example, FDA has issued new guidance documents, improved the dance development process, initiated a reviewer certification program for v FDA reviewers, and enhanced its interactive review process for medical ices.

For FY2012, 36% of FDA's total budget comes from user fees.[49] Medical ice user fee revenue provides about 10% of the FDA medical device and liological health program budget.[50] **Figure 4** presents the total program level FDA's device and radiological health program for FY2002 through 2013 with dollars adjusted for inflation (based on 2005 dollars).

Figure 4 also shows the contribution of medical device user fees, which gan in FY2003, to the device and radiological health program budget, as ell as fees collected for the inspection of mammography facilities under the ammography Quality Standards Act (MQSA), which began fee collection in Y1996. For FY2010, user fees collected under MDUFA funded about 20% of e device review program, while user fees collected under PDUFA funded ver 60% of the drug review program.

User fees are an increasing proportion of FDA's device-related budget, as own in **Table 1**. User fees were 7.1% of FDA's devices and radiological ealth program level budget in FY2002 when MQSA was the sole user fee, nd 14.2% of FDA's devices and radiological health program level budget in Y2012, with both MQSA and medical device user fees being collected by the gency. **Table 1** shows that over the period of FY2003 to FY2012, the amount f user fees more than doubled, while the amount of direct appropriations budget authority) increased at a slower rate.

recommendations to Congress not later than January 15, 2012.[33] Minutes of all negotiation meetings between FDA and industry were required to be posted on the FDA website.

MDUFA Impact on FDA Review Time and Budget

The amount of time it takes FDA to reach a review decision to clear a 510(k) notification or approve a PMA application are measures of how well the agency is meeting the goals defined in the MDUFA agreement between FDA and the medical device industry. The time it takes to review a medical device—total review time—is composed of the time FDA handles the application— FDA time—plus the amount of time the device sponsor or submitter requires to respond to requests by FDA for additional information about the device.

According to CDRH Director Shuren, "FDA has been meeting or exceeding goals agreed to by FDA and industry under MDUFA II for approximately 95% of the submissions we review each year. For example, FDA completes at least 90% of 510(k) reviews within 90 days or less."[34] However, Dr. Shuren noted that these "metrics reflect FDA time only; they do not reflect the time taken by device sponsors to respond to requests for additional information. Overall time to decision—the time that FDA has the application, plus the time the manufacturer spends answering any questions FDA may have—has increased steadily since 2001."[35]

Figure 2 shows that while the amount of time FDA spends reviewing a 510(k) has decreased, the average total days for the review of 510(k)s has been increasing. FDA and GAO have both studied this issue of increasing review time. A 2011 FDA analysis of the reasons behind the increased average total days for the review of 510(k)s found that FDA reviewers needed to ask for additional information—called an AI Letter—from the 510(k) device manufacturer or sponsor due to the poor quality of the original submission.[36] According to FDA, these quality issues involved "the device description, meaning the sponsor either did not provide sufficient information about the device to determine what it was developed to do, or the device description was inconsistent throughout the submission."[37]

Furthermore, FDA concluded that "sponsors' failure to address deficiencies identified in first-round AI Letters are major contributors to the increase in total review times. For example, 65% of the time FDA sent a second-round AI Letter because the sponsor failed to submit information requested in the first AI Letter."[38] The 2011 FDA analysis also found "in some cases, the FDA sent AI Letters for inappropriate reasons, such as asking for additional testing that was outside the scope of what would be required for a 510(k) submission, or asking for supporting documentation that was already covered by a standard government form."[39]

GAO also performed an analysis of FDA performance goals regarding 510(k) device review times and requests for additional information from sponsors.[40] GAO found that although FDA met all medical device performance goals for 510(k)s, the total review time—from submission to final decision—has increased substantially in recent years. Regarding the agency's use of AI Letters, the GAO report notes that "the only alternative to requesting additional information is for FDA to reject the submission."[41] Use of the AI Letter allows the sponsors the opportunity to respond, and although the time to final decision is longer, the application has the opportunity to be approved.

Fiscal Year Receipt Cohorts as of March 11, 2012

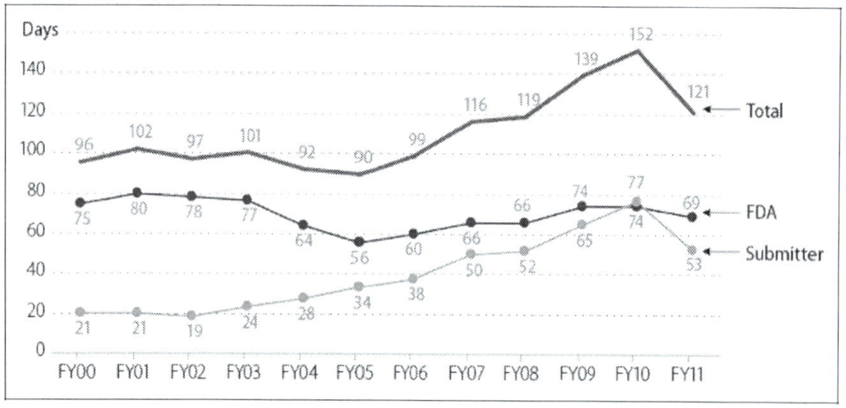

Source: Figure in testimony of CDRH Director Jeffrey Shuren before the Senate HELP Committee, March 29, 2012.

Notes: FDA Days + Submitter Days = Total Time to Decision; times may not add due to rounding. A cohort consists of all 510(k) submissions filed in the same fiscal year. FY2008 through FY2011 cohorts are still open; FY2011 cohort is only 85% closed, and average times will increase.

Figure 2. Average Time to Decision: 510(k)s.

(Non-expedited)

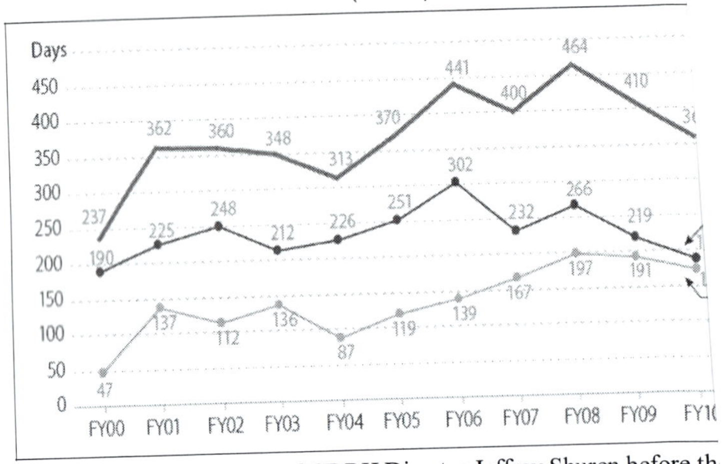

Source: Figure in testimony of CDRH Director Jeffrey Shuren before th
Committee, March 29, 2012.

Notes: FDA Days + Submitter Days = Total Time to Decision; times m
to rounding. Data is for non-expedited PMAs and Panel-Track
Some fiscal year cohorts are still open—data may change. A cohort
submissions of a certain type, in this case PMA, filed in the same f
FY2010, as of January 30, 2012, there were four applications with
the average time to decision will increase as the cohort closes.

Figure 3. Average Time to Decision: PMAs and Panel Track Supplement

Figure 3 provides information on the amount of time F
reviewing non-expedited PMA applications and Panel-Track Sup
device may receive expedited review if it is intended to treat or dia
threatening condition or irreversibly debilitating disease or condi
addresses an unmet need.[42]

CDRH Director Shuren notes that although FDA is spendin
reviewing PMA applications, the average total days for the revie
applications has been increasing since 2004.[43] The February 2012 C
found that for FY2003 through FY2010, FDA met most of the goals
but fell short on most of the goals for expedited PMAs.[44]

The February 2012 GAO report found that FDA review time a
final decision for both types of PMAs were highly variable but
increased during this period.[45]

The February 2012 GAO report also commented on comn
problems between industry and FDA based on interviews with thre
groups about the medical device review process.

ofte
"aft
fro
sub

def
wo
ind
spo
"cr
sub
poi
ind

gu
ne
de

de
ra
fo
FY

be
w
M
F
th
o

s
h
a
F
a
c

Table1. FDA Devices and Radiological Health Program, Fees as a Percentage of Total Program Level (Unadjusted dollars in millions)

Fiscal Year	Budget Authority	MDUFA[a] Fees	MQSA[b] and Other Fees[c]	Total Fees	Total Fees as % of Total Program Level	Total Program Level
2002	$180.0	$0	$13.7	$13.7	7.1%	$193.7
2003	$193.4	$11.1	$12.9	$24.0	11.0%	$217.3
2004[d]	$191.1	na	na	$30.4	13.7%	$221.5
2005	$215.0	$16.4	$13.0	$29.3	12.0%	$244.3
2006	$220.6	$20.7	$13.8	$34.5	13.5%	$255.0
2007	$230.7	$23.3	$13.6	$36.9	13.8%	$267.5
2008	$237.7	$24.3	$13.3	$37.6	13.7%	$275.3
2009	$298.5	$33.3	$13.5	$46.8	13.6%	$345.3
2010	$313.5	$42.7	$13.8	$56.5	15.3%	$370.0
2011	$322.2	$42.0	$14.4	$56.3	14.9%	$378.5
2012	$322.7	$34.2	$19.1	$53.3	14.2%	$376.0
2013	$319.1	$41.4	$26.3	$67.6	17.5%	$386.8

Source: FDA Justification of Estimates for Appropriations Committees documents, FY2004 through FY2013,

a. MDUFA is Medical Device User Fee Act.

b. MQSA is Mammography Quality Standards Act.

c. For FY2013, the Obama Administration proposes a new Field Reinspection fee and a new International Courier User Fee.

d. The FY2006 *Justification* organized data, including Actual data for FY2004, in a format different than other *Justification* documents (it included rent but did not include the Office of Regulatory Affairs). The FY2007 and FY2008 *Justification* documents provided data in consistent format (without rent but included ORA) for FY2004 Budget Authority, Total Fees, and Total Program Level, but did not provide medical device user fees or MQSA amounts. The FY2006 *Justification* provided the following amounts for Actual FY2004 user fees: medical device user fees, $18.245 million; MQSA, $4.039 million; ORA user fees, $9.071 million.

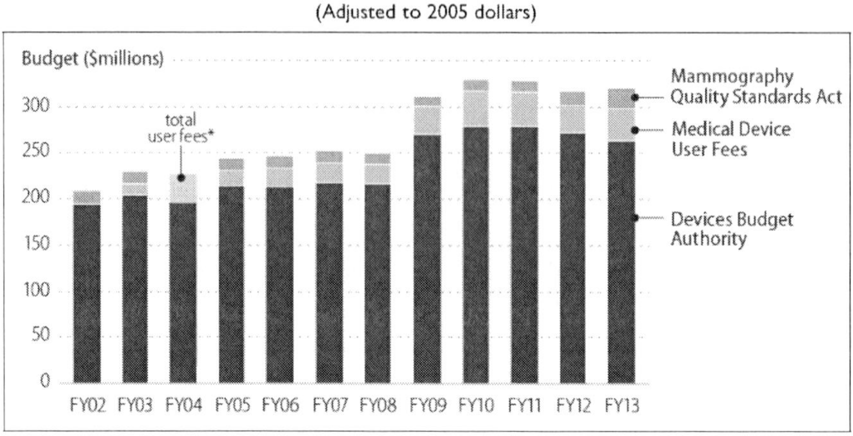

Source: FDA *Justification of Estimates for Appropriations Committees* documents, FY2004 through FY2013.

* Only total user fees were available for FY2004; amounts for medical device user fees and MQSA fees were not identified in the FY2006 *Justification of Estimates for Appropriations Committees*. See **Table 1**.

Notes: Total Program Level = Budget Authority + Medical Device User Fees + MQSA Fees. Data have been adjusted to constant 2005 dollars using "Total Non-Defense" deflators from Office of Management and Budget, *Fiscal Year 2013 Historical Tables, Budget of the U.S. Government*, "Table 10.1, Gross Domestic Product and Deflators Used in the Historical Tables: 1940-2017," pp. 211-212.

Figure 4. Devices and Radiological Health Program Budget, by Funding Source, for FY2002 to FY2013.

MDUFA III Proposal

An initial public meeting on the reauthorization of the medical device user fees was held by FDA on September 14, 2010, after which the negotiation process between FDA and industry began, as well as monthly meetings with other stakeholders.[51] Minutes of the 35 negotiation meetings between FDA and the medical device industry are posted on the agency's website, as are minutes of the 14 monthly meetings with the other stakeholders, such as health care professional associations and patient and consumer advocacy groups.[52]

On February 1, 2012, FDA announced that it had reached "an agreement in principle on proposed recommendations for the third reauthorization of a medical device user fee program."[53] According to a press release on the FDA website, the recommendations would authorize $595 million in user fees collected by the agency from the medical device industry over a five-year period.[54] FDA would be able to hire more than 200 full-time-equivalent workers with this additional funding. In the minutes for the January 31, 2012, negotiation meeting, industry noted "that MDUFA III represents a sizeable increase of 240 FTEs from current levels, FDA should not expect this type of significant resource increase under MDUFA IV."[55] In response, the agency stated that it had "some concerns about how solid a financial footing this agreement establishes, given that there are a lot of uncertainties about how much effort will be required to meet the goals, and that in order to bring the proposal to a level that Industry could agree to, FDA had to take away any margin of error."[56]

On March 14, 2012, the agency posted on its website the draft negotiated package—composed of statutory language and the FDA-industry agreement on performance goals and procedures— referred to as MDUFA III.[57] A public meeting describing the draft was held on March 28, 2012. The 30-day comment period on the draft ended April 16, 2012. Following review of the comments, FDA may revise the recommendation and then is to submit the final package to Congress.

Tables in the appendixes provide additional details on the draft MDUFA III proposal beyond the narrative discussion found below. The tables in **Appendix A** relate to the legislative language and the table in **Appendix B** relates to the FDA-industry agreement on performance goals and procedures.

Draft Legislative Language

The draft legislative language portion of the MDUFA III proposal would change the definition of "establishment subject to a registration fee," increasing the number of establishments paying the fee from 16,000 to about 22,000.[58] It would set the fee amount for a PMA in FY2013 at $248,000. The fee amount for a PMA would gradually rise to $268,443 for FY2017. The establishment fee would be $2,575 in FY2013 and rise to $3,872 for FY2016 and FY2017. Other than the establishment fee, the amount of each type of user fee is set as a percentage of the PMA fee, also called the base fee. The draft proposal would keep the percentages the same as in current law except for the 510(k) fee, which would change from 1.84% of the PMA fee to 2% of the PMA fee. Total fee revenue would be set at $97,722,301 for FY2013 and rise to $130,184,348 for FY2017. The total fees collected over the five-year period FY2013 through FY2017 would be $595 million.

The draft MDUFA III legislative language would adjust the total revenue amounts by a specified inflation adjustment, similar to the adjustment made under PDUFA, and the base fee amount would be adjusted as needed on a uniform proportional basis to generate the inflation-adjusted total revenue amount. After the base fee amounts are adjusted for inflation, the establishment fee amount would be further adjusted as necessary so that the total fee collections for the fiscal year would generate the total adjusted revenue amount. The new adjusted fee amounts would be published in the *Federal Register* 60 days before the start of each fiscal year along with the rationale for adjusting the fee amounts.

The draft legislative language includes a provision that would allow FDA to grant a waiver or reduce fees for a PMA or establishment fee "if the waiver is in the interest of public health." According to the FDA presentation at the March 28, 2012, public meeting, the fee waiver is intended for laboratory developed test (LDT) manufacturers. This provision would sunset at the end of MDUFA III.

The draft proposal includes a requirement that sponsors submit an electronic copy of a PMA, 510(k), and other specified submissions and any supplements to such submissions. The requirement would begin after the issuance of final guidance. The draft legislative language also includes a provision for streamlined hiring of FDA employees. The authority for streamlined hiring would terminate three years after enactment.

Draft Industry-FDA Performance Goals and Procedures for MDUFA III: The Agreement

The agreement begins by stating, "FDA and the industry are committed to protecting and promoting public health by providing timely access to safe and effective medical devices. Nothing in this letter precludes the Agency from protecting the public health by exercising its authority to provide a reasonable assurance of the safety and effectiveness of medical devices."[59] The agreement subsequently describes a number of process improvements that aim to improve FDA's medical device review process, provides revised performance goals and new shared outcome goals, describes infrastructure improvements, and provides for an independent assessment of the device review process.

Process Improvements

In comparison to MDUFA II, the discussion of these topics is greatly expanded and consolidated into one new section of the agreement. FDA will put in place a structured process for managing pre-submissions, providing feedback to applicants via e-mail and a one-hour meeting or teleconference. It will publish guidance on electronic submissions and will clarify submission acceptance criteria. The agency will continue to use interactive review to encourage informal communication with the applicant to facilitate timely completion of the review process. FDA will continue to apply user fees to the guidance document development process, and may apply user fees to delete outdated guidance, note which are under review, and provide a list of prioritized device guidance documents intended to be published within a year. It will work with interested parties to improve the current third-party review program. FDA will implement final guidance on factors to consider when making benefit-risk determinations in device premarket review, including patient tolerance for risk and magnitude of benefit. The agency will propose additional low-risk medical devices to exempt from the 510(k) process. FDA will work with industry to develop a transitional in vitro diagnostics (IVD) approach for the regulation of emerging diagnostics.

Review Performance Goals

The main focus of the agreement is FDA's commitment to completing the review of the various medical device submissions—such as PMA reviews and 510(k) notifications—within specified timeframes in exchange for an industry fee to support the review activity. Performance goals are specified for each type of submission and for FY2013 through FY2017; each goal specifies the percentage of applications FDA will complete along with a given time period. See **Table B-1** and **Table D-1** for further details.

Shared Outcome Goals

This is a new section and was not part of the MDUFA II agreement. The purpose of the programs and initiatives outlined in the agreement is to reduce the average total time to decision for PMAs and 510(k)s. FDA and applicants share the responsibility for achieving this goal. For PMA submissions received beginning in FY2013, the average total time to decision goal for FDA and industry is 395 calendar days; beginning in FY2015, 390 calendar days; and beginning in FY2017, 385 calendar days. For 510(k) submissions received beginning in FY2013, the average total time to decision goal for FDA and industry is 135 calendar days; beginning in FY2015, 130 calendar days; and beginning in FY2017, 124 calendar days.

Infrastructure

User fees will be used to "reduce the ratio of review staff to front line supervisors in the Pre-market review program."[60] FDA will enhance and supplement scientific review capacity by hiring reviewers and using external experts to assist with device application review. FDA will seek to obtain streamlined hiring authority and work with industry to benchmark best practices for employee retention via financial and non-financial means. User fees will supplement (1) management training; (2) MDUFA III training for all staff; (3) Reviewer Certification Program for new CDRH reviewers; and (4) specialized training to provide continuous learning for all staff. FDA will improve its IT system to allow real-time status information on submissions.

Independent Assessment of Review Process Management

By the end of the second quarter of FY2013, FDA will hire a consultant to assess the device application review process. Within six months of award of the contract, a report on recommendations likely to have a significant impact on review time will be published. The final report will be published within one year of contract award date. FDA will publish a corrective action and implementation plan within six months of receipt of each report. The consultant will evaluate FDA's implementation and publish a report no later than February 1, 2016.

Performance Reports

As was the case in MDUFA II, FDA will meet with industry on a quarterly basis to present data and discuss progress in meeting goals. The agreement requires more detailed information to be covered in quarterly reports by CDRH and CBER; specifically, elements to be included are listed for 510(k)s, PMAs, Pre-Submissions, and Investigational Device Exemptions (IDEs).[61] CDRH reports quarterly and CBER reports annually on 11 additional data points. FDA reports annually on nine other topics.

Discretionary Waiver

FDA will seek authority to grant discretionary fee waivers or reduced fees in the interest of public health. Authority for the waiver and reduced fees would expire at the end of MDUFA III. According to the FDA presentation at the March 28, 2012, public meeting, the fee waiver is intended for laboratory developed test (LDT) manufacturers.

Other Potential Issues

In addition to MDUFA III, Congress is considering reauthorization of PDUFA as well as new proposals for a Generic Drug User Fee Act and a Biosimilars User Fee Act. It is likely that these three will be combined with MDUFA III along with a variety of related and unrelated issues. Because of the importance of user fees to FDA's budget, PDUFA and MDUFA are considered to be "must pass" legislation, and Congress has often in the past included language to address a range of other concerns. For example, MDUFA II included provisions about the extent to which FDA can delegate activities to third parties (inspections and the review of premarket notifications); establishment registration requirements (timing and electronic submission); a unique device identification system; and reporting requirements for devices linked to serious injuries or deaths. Provisions that have been mentioned as possibly being included in current legislation containing FDA user fee authorization include the following:

- reauthorization of Best Pharmaceutical for Children Act (BPCA) and Pediatric Research Equity Act (PREA);
- provisions to prevent, avert, or manage drug shortages;
- incentives for antibiotic makers;
- security of the pharmaceutical supply chain;
- less restrictive FDA advisory committee conflict-of-interest waiver policies;
- parity for foreign and domestic manufacturing inspections;
- quicker approval of drugs to treat very rare diseases;
- increased input from patients, hospitals, pharmacists, and others in drug development, review, and postmarket study;
- recall authority for drug products;
- personal-use and commercial drug importation;
- clarification of the least burdensome standard in requesting additional information from sponsors of PMA or 510(k) submissions;
- expanding FDA's authority to require a manufacturer to conduct postmarket surveillance of class II and class III medical devices;
- inclusion of medical devices in the Sentinel Initiative/System;[62]

- extension of the humanitarian device exemption;
- continuation of a demonstration grant program on improving the availability of pediatric devices;
- extension of the third-party review program for 510(k) submissions; and
- limiting the use of a recalled medical device as a predicate in 510(k) submissions.

The House Committee on Energy and Commerce, Subcommittee on Health held a hearing on MDUFA on February 15, 2012, and the Senate Committee on Health, Education, Labor and Pensions held a hearing on FDA user fee agreements on March 29, 2012. The hearing testimony submitted to both the House and Senate by CDRH Director Jeffrey Shuren stated that in FY2010, user fee revenue funded about 20% of the medical device premarket review process; fees collected under MDUFA III would fund about a third of the medical device premarket review process.[63] In contrast, fees collected under PDUFA in FY2010 covered more than 60% of drug review costs. In response to questioning at the Senate hearing, CDRH Director Shuren said if MDUFA reauthorization by Congress has not occurred by early summer, federal regulations require that reduction in force (RIF) notices be sent out in July 2012, giving 60 days' advance notice to about 250 FDA employees that their employment under the MDUFA program would end by September 30, 2012.

The House and Senate committees circulated discussion drafts that contain many of the above listed provisions.[64] CDRH Director Shuren indicated that some of these pending reforms could conflict with what the agency has negotiated with industry in the MDUFA III proposal. "There are several provisions that could have an impact, that could divert resources from implementation of the MDUFA goals and/or that go to issues that were discussed as a part of MDUFA ... that would be counter and would reopen those discussions," according to CDRH Director Shuren.[65] He indicated that proposals regarding device tracking, guidance development, and third-party reviews were of concern, but that "there are many others ... particularly in the House bill."[66] Some proposals are of concern because they would require more agency resources; other proposals were discussed during the user fee negotiations with industry and "taken off the table."[67]

APPENDIX A. PROVISIONS IN FFDCA §737 AND §738

Table A-1. Provisions in Section 737 and 738 of the Federal Food, Drug, and Cosmetic Act Relating to Medical Device User Fees

Main Issue	Current Law	MDUFA III Statutory Language that HHS Submitted to Congress
Section 737. Definitions.		
Definitions	Provides definitions for a number of terms.	Would update the definition of "adjustment factor" and change the definition of "establishment subject to a registration fee," increasing the number paying the fee from 16,000 to 22,000.
Section 738. Authority to Assess and Use Device Fees.		
(a)(1) Types of fees	There are several types of fees and certain exceptions to the collection of such fees.	
(a)(2)(A) PMA, premarket report, supplement, and submission fee, and annual fee for periodic reporting concerning a class III device	A fee is assessed for: premarket application (PMA) premarket report, equal to the PMA fee panel track supplement, 75% of the PMA fee 180-day supplement, 15% of the PMA fee real-time supplement, 7% of the PMA fee 30-day notice, 1.6% of the PMA fee efficacy supplement, equal to the PMA fee premarket notification submission [510(k)], 1.84% of the PMA fee request for classification information, 1.35% of the PMA fee periodic reporting concerning class III device, 3.5% of PMA fee.	Would set fee for 510(k) at 2% of the PMA fee

Table A-1. (Continued)

Main Issue	Current Law			MDUFA III Statutory Language that HHS Submitted to Congress		
(a)(2)(B) Exceptions	Exceptions are made for humanitarian device exemption, PMA for a biologic product licensed for further manufacturing use only, devices sponsored by state or federal government and not intended for commercial distribution, 510(k) reviewed by an accredited third party, and PMAs, premarket reports and 510(k)s if the device is intended solely for a pediatric population, as well as supplements proposing conditions of use for a pediatric population.					
(a)(2)(C)(D) Payment, Refund	The fee is due at the time of submission. Partial or full refunds of fees either may or must occur, depending on certain conditions.					
(a)(3) Annual establishment registration fee	An establishment registration fee is assessed annually. Exceptions are made for an establishment operated by state or federal government entity, and Indian tribes unless the device is intended for commercial distribution.			Would make technical change to date payable.		
(b) Fee amounts	Fees are based on the following amounts which may be adjusted by the Secretary for various reasons:			New (b)(1)-(2). Would change fee amounts and change reasons for adjustment:		
	PMA	Establishment		PMA	Establish.	
	FY2008	$185,000	$1,706	FY2013:	$248,000;	$2,575
	FY2009	$200,725	$1,851	FY2014:	$252,960;	$3,200
	FY2010	$217,787	$2,008	FY2015:	$258,019;	$3,750
	FY2011	$236,298	$2,179	FY2016:	$263,180;	$3,872
	FY2012	$256,384	$2,364	FY2017:	$268,443;	$3,872

Main Issue	Current Law	MDUFA III Statutory Language that HHS Submitted to Congress
(h) Crediting and availability of fees	FY2008 $48,431,000 [FY2013 $95,429,314] FY2009 $52,547,000 [FY2014 $112,171,877] FY2010 $57,014,000 [FY2015 $127,537,959] FY2011 $61,860,000 [FY2016 $129,997,509] FY2012 $67,118,000 [FY2017 $130,328,967] Bracketed amounts in proposal, not current law.	Total revenue amounts, new (b)(3). Would set total fee revenue amounts as follows: FY2013 $97,722,301 FY2014 $112,580,497 FY2015 $125,767,107 FY2016 $129,339,949 FY2017 $130,184,348.
(c)(1) Annual fee setting; in general	The Secretary publishes fee amounts in the Federal Register 60 days before the start of each fiscal year.	Secretary would, 60 days before the start of each fiscal year, establish fees based on amounts specified in subsection (b) and the adjustments in this subsection, and publish such fees and rationale for adjusting fee amounts in the Federal Register.
(c)(2) Adjustment	The Secretary may increase the establishment fee for FY2010 only if the estimate of number of establishments submitting fees for FY2009 is less than 12,250. If the fee for FY2010 is adjusted, fees for FY2011 and FY2012 may be increased by 8.5% over the previous year. The determination and its rationale must be published in the Federal Register.	Inflation adjustment. Would adjust total revenue amounts by a specified inflation adjustment based on the sum of one plus—the average annual change in the cost per FTE position at FDA of all personnel compensation and benefits paid for the first 3 years of the preceding 4 fiscal years, multiplied by 0.60, and the average annual change in the Consumer Price Index (Metro DC, Baltimore, WV. not seasonally adjusted, all items, annual

Table A-1. (Continued)

Main Issue	Current Law	MDUFA III Statutory Language that HHS Submitted to Congress
		index) for the first 3 years of the preceding 4 years of available data multiplied by 0.40. If the sum is less than 1, the sum is considered to be 1; or greater than 1.04, the sum is considered to be 1.04. The base fee amounts in new subsection (b) (2) would be adjusted as needed on a uniform proportional basis to generate the inflation adjusted total revenue amount.
Adjustment To establishment registration base fees	No provision.	New (c) (3). For each fiscal year, after the base fee amounts in new subsection (b)(2) are adjusted for inflation, the base establishment registration fee amounts would be further adjusted as necessary for total fee collections for the fiscal year to generate the total adjusted revenue amount.
(c)(3) Limit	For each fiscal year, the total amount of fees, as adjusted, may not exceed the total costs for the resources allocated for the process for the review of device applications.	Now (c)(4)
(c)(4) Supplement	Secretary may use unobligated carryover balances from fees collected in previous years to ensure sufficient fee revenues are available, so long as there is a certain operating reserve. Not later than 14 days before using these funds, the Secretary must provide	Now (c)(5)

Main Issue	Current Law	MDUFA III Statutory Language that HHS Submitted to Congress
	notice to House and Senate Appropriation Committees, Senate HELP and House Energy and Commerce Committees.	
(d)(e) Small businesses; fee waiver and fee reduction	Secretary may waive the fee for the first premarket review or first premarket report of a product submitted by a small business, defined as an entity that reported less than $30 million in gross receipts or sales in its most recent federal income tax return. If a device company has annual gross receipts or sales of $100 million or less in the most recent federal income tax return for a taxable year, including returns of its affiliates, the device manufacturer is a small business eligible for 75% reduction in fees for PMAs, premarket reports, supplements, and periodic reporting concerning class III devices. Such a device manufacturer is also considered a small business eligible for a reduced rate of 50% for fees regarding 510(k)s, 30-day notices and requests for classification information. Proof of gross sales or receipts may consist of IRS tax documents or qualifying documentation from the taxing authority of the foreign country in which the applicant or affiliate is headquartered.	
Fee waiver or reduction	No provision.	Would allow the Secretary to grant a waiver or reduced fees for a PMA or establishment fee if the waiver is in the interest of public health. Waivers & fee reductions must be less than 2% of total fee revenue for that year. Authority for the waiver and reduced fees ends on October 1, 2017.

Table A-1. (Continued)

Main Issue	Current Law	MDUFA III Statutory Language that HHS Submitted to Congress
(f) Effect of failure to pay fees	PMAs, 510(k), requests for classification, and other submissions for which fees apply will not be accepted if fees are not paid.	
(g) Conditions (Trigger)	Direct appropriations must be more than 1% less than \$205,720,000 multiplied by an adjustment factor, or else the Secretary may not collect user fees and is not required to meet performance goals.	Changes amount to \$280,587,000.
(h) Crediting and availability of fees	The following amounts of user fees are authorized to be appropriated: FY2008 \$48,431,000 FY2009 \$52,547,000 FY2010 \$57,014,000 FY2011 \$61,860,000 FY2012 \$67,118,000 Offset is handled as follows: the amount of fees collected, in the first three fiscal years and estimated for the fourth fiscal year, in excess of the amount specified in appropriations acts is credited to FDA's appropriation account, and the excess subtracted from the amount that would otherwise have been authorized to be collected during the fifth fiscal year.	Would add provision allowing the Secretary to accept early payment of authorized fees. Would authorize to be appropriated for FY2013 through FY2017 fees equal to the total revenue amount as specified under new subsection(b)(3), as adjusted for inflation and offset.
(i) Collection of unpaid fees	Any unpaid fee shall be treated as a claim of the United States Government.	
(j) Written requests for refunds	A sponsor must submit a written request to the Secretary for a refund not later than 180 days after the fee is due.	

Main Issue	Current Law	MDUFA III Statutory Language that HHS Submitted to Congress
(k) Construction	"This section may not be construed to require that" HHS reduce FTE positions of officers, employees, and advisory committee members in other areas to offset those "engaged in the process of the review of device applications."	

Sources: FFDCA §§737-738 (21 U.S.C. §§379i-379j); and FDA, "Draft MDUFA III Legislative Language," dated February 17, 2012, posted on FDA website March 14, 2012, at http://www.fda.gov/downloads/MedicalDevices/NewsEvents/Workshops Conferences/UCM295424.pdf.

Note: Paragraph and subparagraph labeling follows current law.

Table A-2. Provisions in Draft MDUFA III Legislative Language That Would Add Two New Sections to Chapter VII of the Federal Food, Drug, and Cosmetic Act

Main Issue	Provision Included in Draft MDUFA Legislation
Subchapter D—Information and Education Section 74x	Would require that after final guidance is issued, PMA, 510(k), Product Development Protocol, Investigational Device Exemption (IDE), Humanitarian Device Exemption (HDE), and other specified pre-submissions and submissions, and any supplements to such submissions must include an electronic copy.
Subchapter A—General Administrative Provisions Section 7xx Streamlined hiring authority	Would allow the Secretary, without regard to provisions in title 5 U.S.C., to appoint employees to appoint FDA employees to positions related to the process for the review of device applications in order to achieve the performance goals referred to in section 738A(a)(1) as set forth in the Secretary's Commitment Letter. The authority to appoint such employees would terminate three years after the date of enactment.

Source: FDA, "Draft MDUFA III Legislative Language," dated February 17, 2012, posted on FDA website March 14, 2012, at http://www.fda.gov/downloads/MedicalDevices/NewsEvents/WorkshopsConferences/ UCM295424.pdf.

Appendix B. MDUFA III Agreement: Performance Goals and Procedures

Table B-1. Performance Goals and Procedures in Agreement between FDA and Industry Representatives for FY2013 through FY2017 under the Draft MDUFA III

Topic	Draft MDUFA III commitments	Similar language in MDUFA II commitments
I. Process Improvements	Pre-Submissions. FDA will issue draft guidance and final guidance on a new structured process for managing Pre-Submissions. Upon receipt of a Pre-Submission, FDA intends to schedule a one hour meeting or teleconference, if requested. Within 14 days of receipt, FDA will determine if the Pre-Submission meets the definition and notify the applicant if it does not. Three business days prior to meeting, FDA will provide initial feedback via email. FDA and applicant may cancel meeting if no longer needed based on email that will serve as final written feedback. Within 15 days, applicant provides draft minutes including agreements and action items, and FDA edits minutes which become final 15 days after received by applicant. FDA feedback is intended to be final, unless FDA concludes that the feedback does not address important new safety and effectiveness issues.	FDA will make every effort to schedule both informal and formal meetings, both before and during the review process, in a timely manner. These meetings include pre-submission meetings.
	Submission Acceptance Criteria. Prior to implementation, FDA will publish draft and final guidance on electronic submissions and objective criteria for revised "refuse to accept/refuse to file" checklists.	New section.
	Interactive Review. As described in current guidance, FDA will continue to use interactive review to encourage informal communication between agency and applicant to facilitate timely completion of the review process.	FDA will continue to use interactive review process to encourage communication and facilitate review.
	Guidance Document Development. FDA will apply user fees to the guidance document development process, but not to the detriment of meeting the quantitative review timelines and statutory obligations. FDA will update its website, deleting outdated guidance, noting which are under review, and providing a list of prioritized device guidance documents intended to be published within 12 months and other device guidance documents intended to be published as resources permit.	FDA will develop guidance documents to the extent possible without impacting device review time and will post guidance under development for comment.

Topic	Draft MDUFA III commitments	Similar language in MDUFA II commitments
	Third Party Review. FDA will work with interested parties to improve the current program and transparency, but not to the detriment of meeting the quantitative review timelines and statutory obligations.	
	Patient Safety and Risk Tolerance. FDA will fully implement final guidance on factors to consider when making benefit-risk determinations in device premarket review, including patient tolerance for risk, magnitude of benefit, and availability of other treatments or diagnostic tests.	New section.
	Low Risk Medical Device Exemptions. By the end of FY2013, FDA will propose additional low risk medical devices to exempt from the 510(k) process and intends to issue a final rule within 2 years exempting additional low risk devices from 510(k).	New section.
	Emerging Diagnostics. FDA will work with industry to develop a transitional in vitro diagnostics (IVD) approach for the regulation of emerging diagnostics.	To facilitate IVD development, FDA will explore ways to clarify the regulatory requirements by issuing guidance as well as 5 other specified activities.
II. Review performance goals	PMA, Panel-Track Supplements, and Premarket Report Applications. Performance goals apply to all PMAs, Panel-Track Supplements, and Premarket Report Applications including those that are priority review (previously referred to as expedited). FDA will communicate with applicant on status of application within 15 days of receipt. For submissions that do not require Advisory Committee input, FDA will issue a MDUFA decision within 180 FDA Days for: 70% of submissions received in FY2013; 80% of submissions received in FY2014 and FY2015; and 90% of submissions received in FY2016 and FY2017. For submissions that require Advisory Committee input, FDA will issue a MDUFA decision within 320 FDA Days for: 50% of submissions received in FY2013; 70% of submissions received in FY2014; 80% of submissions received in FY2015 and FY2016; and 90% of submissions received in FY2017. For all PMAs that do not reach a MDUFA decision by 20 days after the FDA Day goal, FDA will provide written feedback to the applicant including all outstanding issues preventing FDA from reaching a decision.	FDA will issue a decision for 60% of non-expedited filed submissions within 180 days, and for 90% within 295 days. FDA will issue a decision for 50% of expedited filed submissions within 180 days and for 90% within 280 days.

Table B-1. (Continued)

Topic	Draft MDUFA III commitments	Similar language in MDUFA II commitments
	180-Day PMA Supplements. FDA will communicate with applicant within 90 days of receipt of the submission for: 65% of submissions received in FY2013; 75% of submissions received in FY2014; 85% of submissions received in FY2015; and 95% of submissions received in FY2016 through FY2017. FDA will issue a MDUFA decision within 180 FDA Days for: 85% of submissions received in FY2013; 90% of submissions received in FY2014 and FY2015; and 95% of submissions received in FY2016 through FY2017.	FDA will issue a decision for 85% within 180 days and for 95% within 210 days.
	Real-Time PMA Supplements. FDA will issue a MDUFA decision within 90 FDA Days for: 90% of such submissions received in FY2013 and FY2014; and 95% of such submissions received in FY2015 through FY2017.	FDA will issue a decision for 80% within 60 days, and for 90% within 90 days.
	510(k) Submissions. FDA will communicate with applicant on status of application within 15 days of receipt. For submissions received in FY2013, FDA will issue a MDUFA decision for 91% of 510(k) submissions within 90 FDA Days. For submissions received in FY2014, FDA will issue a MDUFA decision for 93% of 510(k) submissions within 90 FDA Days. For submissions received in FY2015 through FY2017, FDA will issue a MDUFA decision for 95% of 510(k) submissions within 90 FDA Days. For all 510(k)s that do not reach a MDUFA decision within 100 FDA Days, FDA will provide written feedback to the applicant including all outstanding issues preventing FDA from reaching a decision.	FDA will issue a decision for 90% of 510(k)s within 90 days, and for 98% within 150 days.
	CLIA Waiver by Application. During the pre-submission process, if the applicant informs FDA that it plans to submit a dual submission (510(k) and CLIA Waiver application), FDA will issue a decision for 90% of such applications within 210 FDA days. For "CLIA Waiver by Application" submissions FDA will issue a MDUFA decision: for 95% of the applications that do not require Advisory Committee input within 180 FDA days; for 95% of the applications that require Advisory Committee input within 330 FDA days. FDA will issue guidance regarding review and management expectations to provide greater transparency throughout the entire submission process.	New section.
	Biologics Licensing Applications (BLAs). FDA will review and act on standard original BLA submissions within 10 months of receipt for 90% of submissions. FDA will review and act on priority original BLA submissions within 6 months of receipt for 90% of	90% of BLAs in 10 months. 90% of BLA supplements in 10 months.

Topic	Draft MDUFA III commitments	Similar language in MDUFA II commitments
	submissions. FDA will review and act on standard BLA efficacy supplement submissions within 10 months of receipt for 90% of submissions. FDA will review and act on priority BLA efficacy supplement submissions within 6 months of receipt for 90% of submissions. FDA will review and act on Class 1 original BLA and BLA efficacy supplement resubmissions within 2 months of receipt for 90% of submissions. FDA will review and act on Class 2 original BLA and BLA efficacy supplement resubmissions within 6 months of receipt for 90% of submissions. FDA will review and act on BLA manufacturing supplements requiring prior approval within 4 months of receipt for 90% of submissions.	90% of BLA resubmissions and BLA supplement resubmissions in two months
III. Shared Outcome Goal	Process improvements in the agreement are intended to reduce the average Total Time to Decision for PMAs and 510(k)s. FDA and applicants share the responsibility for achieving this goal. PMA. For submissions received beginning in FY2013, the average Total Time to Decision goal for FDA and industry is 395 calendar days; beginning in FY2015, 390 calendar days; beginning in FY2017, 385 calendar days. 510(k). For submissions received beginning in FY2013, the average Total Time to Decision goal for FDA and industry is 135 calendar days; beginning in FY2015, 130 calendar days; beginning in FY2017, 124 calendar days.	New section.
IV. Infrastructure	Scientific and Regulatory Review Capacity. User fees will be used to reduce the ratio of review staff to supervisors and to enhance and supplement scientific review capacity by hiring reviewers and leveraging external experts needed to assist with device application review. FDA will seek to obtain streamlined hiring authority and work with industry to benchmark best practices for retaining employees (both financial and non-financial).	New section.
	Training. FDA will hold at least two medical device Vendor Days each year. User fees will supplement the following: management training; MDUFA III train for all staff; Reviewer Certification Program for new reviewers; specialized training to provide continuous learning for all staff.	FDA will apply user fees to support reviewer training that is related to the process for the review of devices, including training to enhance scientific expertise.
	Tracking System. IT system will be improved to allow real-time status information for submissions.	New section.

Table B-1. (Continued)

Topic	Draft MDUFA III commitments	Similar language in MDUFA II commitments
V. Independent Assessment of Review Process Management	By the end of the 2nd quarter of FY2013, FDA will award a contract to assess the device application review process. Within 6 months of award, a report on recommendations likely to have a significant impact on review time will be published; final report will be published within 1 year of contract award. FDA will publish an implementation plan within 6 months of receipt of each report. The contractor will evaluate FDA's implementation and publish a report no later than February 1, 2016.	New section.
VI. Performance Reports	Information to be covered in quarterly reports by CDRH and CBER is listed for: 510(k)s, PMAs; Pre-Submissions; and, IDEs. CDRH reports quarterly and CBER reports annually on 11 data points such as: NSE decisions for 510(k)s; withdrawls of 510(k)s and PMAs; not approvable decisions for PMAs; other noteworthy issues like rates of AI letters; number of submissions that missed goals; new draft and final guidance; fee collection summary; independent assessment implementation plan status; number of discretionary fee waivers. FDA reports annually on nine topics such as: use of fees for enhanced scientific review capacity; number of Premarket Report Submissions; summary of training courses; shared outcome goal performance; 510(k) submissions; PMA submissions; DeNovo classification petitions; CLIA waiver applications.	FDA reports quarterly on progress toward attaining quantitative goals. For all submission types, FDA will track total time from receipt to final decision. FDA provides annually review performance data by branch (grouped by subject), indicating the shortest and longest average review times for 510(k)s, 180-day supplements, and real- time supplements.
VII. Discretionary Waiver	FDA will seek authority to grant discretionary fee waivers or reduced fees in the interest of public health. Authority for the waiver and reduced fees expires at the end of MDUFA III.	New section.
VIII. Definitions and explanations of terms	Total Time to Decision is the number of calendar days from the date to receipt or filed submission to a MDUFA decision. The average Total Time to Decision for 510(k) submissions is calculated as the trimmed mean of Total Times to Decision for 510(k) submissions within a closed cohort, excluding the highest 2% and the lowest 2% of values. A cohort is closed when 99% of the accepted submissions have reached a decision. A cohort consists of all submissions of a certain type, in this case 510(k), filed in the same fiscal year.	The following terms were defined: FDA Decision; Expedited Review; PMA Modules; 180-Day PMA Supplements; and, Real-Time Supplements.

Topic	Draft MDUFA III commitments	Similar language in MDUFA II commitments
	The average Total Time to Decision for PMA applications is calculated as the three-year rolling average of the annual Total Times to Decision for applications (for example, for FY2015, the average Total Time to Decision for PMA applications would be the average of FY2013 through FY2015) within a closed cohort, excluding the highest 5% and the lowest 5% of values. A cohort is closed when 95% of the applications have reached a decision. A cohort consists of all submissions of a certain type, in this case PMA, filed in the same fiscal year. Other terms that are defined: Applicant; Electronic Copy; FDA Days; MDUFA decisions; Pre-Submission; and, Substantive Interaction. Three BLA-related definitions are also provided: Review and act on; Class 1 resubmitted applications; and, Class 2 resubmitted applications.	

Source: FDA, "Draft MDUFA III Commitment Letter," dated February 17, 2012, and posted on FDA website March 14, 2012, at http://www.fda.gov/downloads/MedicalDevices/NewsEvents/WorkshopsConferences/UCM295454.pdf. Document is referred to, at times, as the Commitment Letter or the Agreement; and FDA, "MDUFA 2007 Commitment Letter," dated September 27, 2007, and posted on FDA website at http://www.fda.gov/MedicalDevices/DeviceRegulationandGuidance/Overview/MedicalDeviceUserFeeandModernizationActMDUFMA/default.htm.

Note: Topic numbering corresponds to the ordering in draft MDUFA III Agreement; these are usually different from the MDUFA II (2007) numbering.

Appendix C. MDUFMA and MDUFA: Fees and Performance Goals

Table C-1. MDUFMA/MDUFA 2007 Fee Schedule, FY2007-FY2012

Fees Structure	MDUFMA	MDUFA 2007				
	2007	2008	2009	2010	2011	2012
Application Fees						
PMA (i.e., *base fee*)	$281,600	$185,000	$200,725	$217,787	$236,298	$256,384
Small Business[a]	$107,008	$46,250	$50,181	$54,447	$59,075	$64,096
Panel Track Supplement[b]	$281,600	$138,750	$150,544	$163,340	$177,224	$192,288
Small Business[a]	$107,008	$34,688	$37,636	$40,835	$44,306	$48,072
180-Day Supplement[c]	$60,544	$27,750	$30,109	$32,668	$35,445	$38,458
Small Business[a]	$23,007	$6,938	$7,527	$8,167	$8,861	$9,614
Real Time Supplement[d]	$20,275	$12,950	$14,051	$15,245	$16,541	$17,947
Small Business[a]	$7,705	$3,237	$3,512	$3,810	$4,134	$4,485
510(k)	$4,158	$3,404	$3,693	$4,007	$4,348	$4,717
Small Business[a]	$3,326	$1,702	$1,847	$2,004	$2,174	$2,359
30-Day Notice[e]		$2,960	$3,212	$3,485	$3,781	$4,102
Small Business[a]		$1,480	$1,606	$1,742	$1,890	$2,051
513(g)[f]		$2,498	$2,710	$2,940	$3,190	$3,461
Small Business[a]		$1,249	$1,355	$1,470	$1,595	$1,731
Product Fee						
Annual Fee for Periodic Report.		$6,475	$7,025	$7,623	$8,270	$8,973
Small Business[a]		$1,619	$1,756	$1,906	$2,068	$2,243

Fees Structure	MDUFMA	MDUFA 2007				
	2007	2008	2009	2010	2011	2012
Establishment Fee						
Establishment Registration		$1,706	$1,851	$2,008	$2,179	$2,364

Source: FDA, *Medical Devices: Proposed Industry User Fee Schedule for MDUFMA II*, March 3, 2009, accessed on January 31, 2012, http://www.fda.gov/MedicalDevices/DeviceRegulationandGuidance/Overview/MedicalDeviceUserFeeandModernizationAct MDUFMA/ucm109319.htm.

a. Small Business—indicates the reduced small business fee associated with the item listed above.

b. Panel-Track Supplement—manufacturer requests approval of a significant change in the design or performance of a device approved via the PMA pathway; significant amount of clinical data evaluated.

c. 180-Day PMA Supplement—manufacturer requests approval of a change in aspects of an approved device, such as its design, specifications, or labeling; new clinical data not required or only limited clinical data.

d. Real-Time PMA Supplement—manufacturer requests approval for a minor change to an approved device, such as a minor change in the design or labeling.

e. 30-Day Notice—manufacturer requests permission to make modifications to manufacturing procedures or methods of manufacture affecting the safety and effectiveness of the device.

f. 513(g)—manufacturer requests information on the classification of a device.

APPENDIX D. MDUFA III PERFORMANCE GOALS

Table D-1. Summary of Performance Goals per February 7, 2012, Agreement

Submission Type		2007	2008-2012	2013-2017 (01/31/2012 Agreement) - all in FDA Days except Average Total				
		End of MDUFMA I	MDUFA II	FY13	FY14	FY15	FY16	FY17
510(k)	Tier I	80% in 90 days	90% in 90 days	91% in 90 days	93% in 90 days	95% in 90 days	95% in 90 days	95% in 90 days
	Tier 2	N.A.	98% in 150 days					
	Cycle	90% in 75 days	N.A.	N.A.	N.A.	N.A.	N.A.	N.A.
	Interaction	N.A.	N.A.	65% in 60 days	75% in 60 days	85% in 60 days	95% in 60 days	95% in 60 days
	Average Total Time	N.A.	N.A.	135 days	135 days	130 days	130 days	124 days
180 Day PMA Supplement	Tier 1	90% in 180 days	85% in 180 days	85% in 180 days	90% in 180 days	90% in 180 days	95% in 180 days	95% in 180 days
	Tier 2	N.A.	95% in210 days					
	Cycle	90% in 120 days	N.A.	N.A.	N.A.	N.A.	N.A.	N.A.
	Interaction	N.A.	N.A.	65% in 90 days	75% in 90 days	85% in 90 days	95% in 90 days	95% in 90 days
Original PMAs & Panel Track Supplements		Tier 1 - 50% in 180 days	Tier 1 - 60% in 180 days	No Panel - 70% in 180 days	No Panel - 80% in 180 days	No Panel - 80% in 180 days	No Panel - % in 180 days	No Panel - 0% in 180 days
		Tier 2 -90% in 320 days	Tier 2 - 90% in 295 days	With Panel - 50% in 320 days	With Panel - 70% in 320 days	With Panel - 80% in 320 days	With Panel - 80% in 320 days	With Panel - 90% in 320 days

Submission Type		2007	2008-2012	2013-2017 (01/31/2012 Agreement) - all in FDA Days except Average Total				
		End of MDUFMA I	MDUFA II	FY13	FY14	FY15	FY16	FY17
	Cycle	75% in 150 days	N.A.	N.A.	N.A.	N.A.	N.A.	N.A.
	Interaction	N.A.	N.A.	65% in 90 days	75% in 90 days	85% in 90 days	95% in 90 days	95% in 90 days
	Average Total Time	N.A.	N.A.	395 days	395 days	390 days	390 days	385 days
Expedited PMAs	**Tier 1**	90% in 300 days	50% in 180 days	Included with	Included with	Included with	Included with	Included with
	Tier 2	N.A.	90% in 280 days	"Original PMAs"	"Original PMAs"	"Original PMAs"	"Original PMAs"	"Original PMAs"
	Cycle	70% in 120 days	N.A.	90% in 90 days	90% in 90 days	95% in 90 days	95% in 90 days	95% in 90 days
Real Time PMA Supplements	**Tier 1**	N.A.	80% in 60 days	90% in 210 days	95% in 180 days	95% in 180 days	95% in 180 days	90% in 90 days
	Tier 2	N.A.	90% in 90 days	90% in 180 days	95% in 330 days	95% in 330 days	95% in 330 days	95% in 330 days
CLIA Waiver Applications	**Dual CLIA/510(k)**	N.A.	N.A.	90% in 210 days	90% in 210 days	90% in 210 days	90% in 210 days	90% in 210 days
	CLIA –no panel	N.A.	N.A.	95% in 180 days	95% in 180 days	95% in 180 days	95% in 180 days	95% in 180 days
	CLIA –with panel	N.A.	N.A.	95% in 330 days	95% in 330 days	95% in 330 days	95% in 330 days	95% in 330 days

Source: FDA, MDUFA Reauthorization Public Meeting, Slide 17, March 28, 2012.

Note: N.A. = Not Applicable.

APPENDIX E. ACRONYMS USED IN THIS REPORT

510(k)	Premarket Notification
513(g)	Request for Information About Device Classification
BLA	Biologics License Application
CBER	Center for Biologics Evaluation and Research
CDRH	Center for Devices and Radiological Health
CLIA	Clinical Laboratory Improvement Amendments
FDA	United States Food and Drug Administration
FFDCA	Federal Food, Drug, and Cosmetic Act (21 U.S.C. Chapter 9)
FTE	Full Time Equivalent Employee
GAO	Government Accountability Office (formerly General Accounting Office)
HDE	Humanitarian Device Exemption
HELP	Senate Health, Education, Labor and Pensions Committee
HHS	United States Department of Health and Human Services
IDE	Investigational Device Exemption
MDTCA	Medical Device Technical Corrections Act
MDUFMA	Medical Device User Fee and Modernization Act
MDUFA II	Medical Device User Fee Amendments of 2007
MDUFSA	Medical Device User Fee Stabilization Act of 2005
MQSA	Mammography Quality Standards Act
NSE	Non-Substantial Equivalence
PDP	Product Development Protocol
PDUFA	Prescription Drug User Fee Act
PL	Public Law
PMA	Premarket Approval
RIF	Reduction in Force
SE	Substantial Equivalence
SUD	Single-Use Device
USC	United States Code

End Notes

[1] MDUFMA (P.L. 107-250) added Sections 737 and 738 to the Federal Food, Drug and Cosmetic Act (FFDCA) [21 USC 379i and 379j]. MDUFMA was amended twice by the Medical Device Technical Corrections Act of 2004 (MDTCA; P.L. 108-214) and the Medical Device User Fee Stabilization Act of 2005 (MDUFSA; P.L. 109-43).

[2] FDA, Medical Devices, "Is the Product a Medical Device," at http://www.fda.gov/medicaldevices/deviceregulationandguidance/overview/classifyyourdevice/ucm051512.htm.

[3] Another center, the Center for Biologics Evaluation and Research (CBER), regulates devices associated with blood collection and processing procedures, cellular products, and tissues. For more information, see CRS Report R42130, *FDA Regulation of Medical Devices*, by Judith A. Johnson.

[4] These reports are listed in Institute of Medicine (IOM), *Medical Devices and the Public's Health: The FDA 510(k) Clearance Process at 35 Years*, Washington, DC, July 2011, p. 30, http://www.iom.edu/Reports/2011/Medical-Devices-and-the-Publics-Health-The-FDA-510k-Clearance-Process-at-35-Years.aspx.

[5] PDUFA came about following negotiations among the FDA (under Commissioner David Kessler), the drug industry, and key congressional committee Members and staff. The aim of the negotiations was "getting enough qualified doctors onto the FDA staff to carry out drug reviews, and getting the company staffs to cooperate in meeting higher standards. The solution that emerged was one intended to bypass the anachronistic and unreliable congressional system that always underfinanced the FDA." Phillip J. Hilts, *Protecting America's Health* (New York: Alfred A. Knopf, 2003), p. 278. Other key features of PDUFA include ensuring that the user fee revenue would not go to general funds but could be spent only on the drug review program, a sunset provision ensuring the user fee program would be reevaluated every five years, and "an implicit contract by Congress not to exploit the availability of the user fee monies and then reduce FDA appropriations for drug review-related purposes." Daniel Carpenter, *Reputation and Power: Organizational Image and Pharmaceutical Regulation at the FDA* (Princeton, NJ: Princeton University Press, 2010), pp. 459-460.

[6] See CRS Report R42366, *Prescription Drug User Fee Act (PDUFA): Issues for Reauthorization (PDUFA V) in 2012*, by Susan Thaul, and CRS Report RL34459, *Animal Drug User Fee Programs*, by Sarah A. Lister.

[7] MDUFA was enacted as Title II of the Food and Drug Administration Amendments Act of 2007 (FDAAA; P.L. 110-85). See CRS Report RL34465, *FDA Amendments Act of 2007 (P.L. 110-85)*, by Erin D. Williams and Susan Thaul.

[8] Food and Drug Administration, "FDA and Industry reach agreement in principle on medical device user fees," press release, February 1, 2012, http://www.fda.gov/NewsEvents/Newsroom/PressAnnouncements/ucm289828.htm. FDA and industry missed the January 15, 2012, statutory deadline for transmitting the MDUFA III package to Congress, delaying the reauthorization process and possibly jeopardizing completion before the medical device user fee program sunsets on September 30, 2012.

[9] FDA, "Draft MDUFA III Commitment Letter," dated February 17, 2012, and posted on FDA website March 14, 2012, at http://www.fda.gov/downloads/MedicalDevices/NewsEvents/WorkshopsConferences/UCM295454.pdf. Document is referred to, at times, as the Commitment Letter or the Agreement. FDA, draft statutory language dated February 17, 2012, and posted at http://www.fda.gov/downloads/MedicalDevices/NewsEvents/WorkshopsConferences/UCM295424.pdf.

[10] Novel devices lacking a legally marketed predicate are automatically designated Class III. FFDCA Section 513(f) established an expedited mechanism for reclassifying these devices based on risk, reducing the regulatory burden on manufacturers. The de novo 510(k), though requiring more data than a traditional 510(k), often requires less information than a PMA application. For more information on device classification and the FDA review process, see CRS Report R42130, *FDA Regulation of Medical Devices*, by Judith A. Johnson.

[11] U.S. Congress, Senate Special Committee on Aging, A Delicate Balance: FDA and the Reform of the Medical Device Approval Process, Testimony of William Maisel, Deputy Center Director for Science, FDA/CDRH, 112th Cong., 1st sess., April 13, 2011.

[12] U.S. Congress, House Committee on Energy and Commerce, Subcommittee on Health, *Reauthorization of MDUFA: What it means for jobs, innovation and patients*, Statement of Jeffrey Shuren, CDRH Director, FDA, 112th Cong., 2nd sess., February 15, 2012; and U.S. Congress, Senate Committee on Health, Education, Labor and Pensions, *FDA User Fee Agreements*, Statement of Jeffrey Shuren, CDRH Director, FDA, 112th Cong., 2nd sess., March 29, 2012.

[13] Ibid.

[14] FFDCA 738(a)(2)(A).

[15] FDA, "Medical Device User Fee and Modernization Act; Public Meeting," 72 *Federal Register* 19528, April 18, 2007.

[16] FDA, "Medical Device User Fee and Modernization Act; Public Meeting," 72 *Federal Register* 19528, April 18, 2007.

[17] FFDCA 738(a)(2)(A)

[18] FFDCA 738(b).

[19] FDA, "Medical Device User Fee and Modernization Act; Public Meeting," 72 *Federal Register* 19528, April 18, 2007. Under MDUFMA, base fees increased by 34% from FY2003 to FY2004, by 15.7% from FY2004 to FY2005, and by 8.5% from FY2005 to FY2006 and FY2006 to FY2007.

[20] The HHS Secretary had the authority to increase the establishment fee by up to an additional 8.5% (over the annual 8.5% increase) in FY2010 if fewer than 12,250 establishments paid the fee in FY2009. This measure was designed to ensure that the establishment fees were 45% of total fees, ensuring that FDA had a stable funding base from user fees.

[21] FFDCA 738(a)(2)(B); 21 USC 379j(a)(2)(b).

[22] FFDCA 738(a)(2)(B)(i). HDE is intended to encourage the development of devices that aid in the treatment and diagnosis of diseases or conditions that affect fewer than 4,000 individuals in the United States per year. FFDCA 520(m); 21 USC 360j(m). The research and development costs of such devices could exceed the market returns for products that address diseases or conditions affecting small patient populations.

[23] FFDCA 738(a)(2)(B)(v)

[24] FFDCA 738(a)(2)(B)(ii); FFDCA 738(a)(3)(A)

[25] FFDCA 523.

[26] FFDCA 738(a)(2)(B)(iv).

[27] FFDCA 738(d),(e); 21 USC 379j(d),(e).

[28] FDA, "Medical Device User Fee and Modernization Act; Public Meeting," 72 *Federal Register* 19528, April 18, 2007.

[29] FFCCA 738(d); 21 USC 379j(d).

[30] FFDCA 738(g).

[31] Emphasis added. FFDCA 738(h)(2)(A)(ii). The law specifically defines "costs of resources allocated for the process for the review of device applications" and what activities are considered part of the "*process for the review of device applications*." For example, costs include management of information and activities associated with the process for review include inspections of manufacturing establishments. [Emphasis added. FFDCA 737(8)-(9).] The process for review of device applications focuses solely on activities involved in premarket approval, with one exception: the evaluation of postmarket studies that are required as a condition of approval of certain premarket applications or reports. [FFDCA 737(8)(J).]

[32] FFDCA 738A(b)

[33] FFDCA 738A(b)(5).

[34] U.S. Congress, House Committee on Energy and Commerce, Subcommittee on Health, *Reauthorization of MDUFA: What it means for jobs, innovation and patients*, Statement of Jeffrey Shuren, CDRH Director, FDA, 112th Cong., 2nd sess., February 15, 2012; and, U.S. Congress, Senate Committee on Health, Education, Labor and Pensions, *FDA User Fee*

Agreements, Statement of Jeffrey Shuren, CDRH Director, FDA, 112th Cong., 2nd sess., March 29, 2012.

[35] Ibid.

[36] FDA/CDRH, *Analysis of Premarket Review Times Under the 510(k) Program*, July 2011, at http://www.fda.gov/downloads/AboutFDA/CentersOffices/OfficeofMedicalProductsandTobacco/CDRH/CDRHReports/UCM263386.pdf.

[37] Ibid., p. 3. Page 15 of the 2011 FDA/CDRH 510(k) report provides more detail on these deficiencies: "(i) the sponsor did not submit required information without justification – such information includes supporting data required under current guidance or performance data that FDA consistently requires for certain device types; (ii) the sponsor failed to identify a predicate; or (iii) the sponsor employed different device descriptions or indications for use for the subject device throughout its submission. In all of these cases, FDA could not reach a substantial equivalence determination without the sponsor providing additional information or rectifying deficiencies in the submission."

[38] Ibid., p. 15.

[39] Ibid., p. 7. Two separate analyses of AI Letters were conducted: one to assess incoming submission quality (Cohort 1) and one to assess the drivers of the increasing numbers of review cycles (Cohort 2). On page 3 of the July 2011 *Analysis of Premarket Review Times Under the 510(k) Program* report, FDA states that it analyzed AI letters "to determine how often the questions that were asked were appropriate or inappropriate, i.e. were the AI Letters justified or did the reviewer ask for information or data that were not permissible as a matter of federal law or FDA policy, or unnecessary to make an SE [substantially equivalent] determination. Results from Cohort 1 showed that reviewers asked for data that had not previously been requested for particular device types 12% of the time. Of those requests, 4% were appropriate, and 8% were inappropriate. Results of the first-round AI Letters from Cohort 2 showed that reviewers asked for appropriate data that had not previously been requested for particular device types 4% of the time, and 2% of the time those requests were inappropriate."

[40] U.S. Government Accountability Office, *Medical Devices: FDA Has Met Most Performance Goals but Device Reviews Are Taking Longer*, GAO-12-418, February 2012, http://www.gao.gov/products/GAO-12-418.

[41] Ibid., p. 16.

[42] FDA Guidance, Expedited Review of Premarket Submissions for Devices, February 29, 2008, p. 3, at http://www.fda.gov/downloads/MedicalDevices/DeviceRegulationandGuidance/GuidanceDocuments/ucm089698.pdf.

[43] U.S. Congress, House Committee on Energy and Commerce, Subcommittee on Health, *Reauthorization of MDUFA: What it means for jobs, innovation and patients*, Statement of Jeffrey Shuren, CDRH Director, FDA, 112th Cong., 2nd sess., February 15, 2012; and, Senate Committee on Health, Education, Labor and Pensions, *FDA User Fee Agreements*, Statement of Jeffrey Shuren, CDRH Director, FDA, 112th Cong., 2nd sess., March 29, 2012.

[44] Ibid., p. 20.

[45] U.S. Government Accountability Office, *Medical Devices: FDA Has Met Most Performance Goals but Device Reviews Are Taking Longer*, GAO-12-418, February 2012, p. 20, http://www.gao.gov/products/GAO-12-418.

[46] Ibid., p. 34.

[47] Ibid.

[48] Ibid., p. 35.

[49] In addition to medical device user fees, Congress has authorized user fees for prescription drugs, animal drugs, animal generic drugs, tobacco products, mammography, color and export certification, and, most recently, several food-related programs.

[50] Of the $57.6 million in medical device user fees for FY2012, 60% goes to the devices and radiological health program (funding 221 full-time equivalent employees [FTEs]), 20% to the biologics program (29 FTEs), and the remaining 20% to rent and FDA headquarters (21

FTEs). Data from Department of Health and Human Services (HHS), *Fiscal Year 2013 Food and Drug Administration: Justification of Estimates for Appropriations Committees*, February2012, p. 94.

[51] FDA, Public Workshop: Medical Device User Fee Program Public Meeting, September 14, 2010, at http://www.fda.gov/MedicalDevices/NewsEvents/WorkshopsConferences/ ucm 218250.htm.

[52] FDA, Medical Devices, MDUFA Meetings at http://www.fda.gov/MedicalDevices/ DeviceRegulationandGuidance/Overview/MedicalDeviceUserFeeandModernizationActMD UFMA/ucm236902.htm.

[53] Food and Drug Administration, "FDA and Industry reach agreement in principle on medical device user fees," press release, February 1, 2012, http://www.fda.gov/NewsEvents/ Newsroom/PressAnnouncements/ucm289828.htm.

[54] Ibid.

[55] FDA, Minutes From Negotiation Meeting on MDUFA III Reauthorization, January 31, 2012, at http://www.fda.gov/MedicalDevices/DeviceRegulationandGuidance/Overview/Medical DeviceUserFeeandModernizationActMDUFMA/ ucm289824.htm.

[56] Ibid.

[57] FDA, draft statutory language dated February 17, 2012, and posted at http://www.fda.gov/ downloads/MedicalDevices/NewsEvents/WorkshopsConferences/UCM295424.pdf . FDA, "Draft MDUFA III Commitment Letter," dated February 17, 2012, and posted on FDA website March 14, 2012, at http://www.fda.gov/downloads/MedicalDevices/NewsEvents/ WorkshopsConferences/UCM295454.pdf. Document is referred to, at times, as the Commitment Letter or the Agreement.

[58] FDA, MDUFA Reauthorization Public Meeting, March 28, 2012.

[59] FDA, "Draft MDUFA III Commitment Letter," dated February 17, 2012, and posted on FDA website March 14, 2012, at http://www.fda.gov/downloads/MedicalDevices/NewsEvents/ WorkshopsConferences/UCM295454.pdf.

[60] Ibid., p. 12.

[61] An IDE allows an unapproved device (most commonly an invasive or life-sustaining device) to be used in a clinical study to collect the data required to support a PMA submission.

[62] A national electronic system under development that would transform FDA's ability to track the safety of drugs, biologics, and medical devices once they reach the market. FDA launched the Sentinel Initiative in May 2008; once completed, it would be called the Sentinel System. For more information, see http://www.fda.gov/safety/FDAsSentinel Initiative/ucm2007250.htm.

[63] U.S. Congress, House Committee on Energy and Commerce, Subcommittee on Health, *Reauthorization of MDUFA: What it means for jobs, innovation and patients*, Statement of Jeffrey Shuren, CDRH Director, FDA, 112th Cong., 2nd sess., February 15, 2012; and, U.S. Congress, Senate Committee on Health, Education, Labor and Pensions, *FDA User Fee Agreements*, Statement of Jeffrey Shuren, CDRH Director, FDA, 112th Cong., 2nd sess., March 29, 2012.

[64] The draft Senate bill that contains provisions related to the regulation of medical devices can be found at http://www.help.senate.gov/imo/media/audio/031612_Device_DRAFT_ TAM1 2069.pdf. The draft House bill containing both drug and medical device regulation can be found at http://insidehealthpolicy.com/iwpfile.html?file=mar2012% 2Fhe03132012_fee.pdf.

[65] Alaina Busch, "FDA Official: Guidance, Tracking Among Device Bills Clashing With Fee Pact," *InsideHealthPolicy.com*, March 28, 2012.

[66] Ibid.

[67] Ibid.

In: Medical Devices and the FDA
Editors: Gil Frazier and Brady Malone ISBN: 978-1-62257-674-6
© 2013 Nova Science Publishers, Inc.

Chapter 3

RIEGEL V. MEDTRONIC, INC.: FEDERAL PREEMPTION OF STATE TORT LAW REGARDING MEDICAL DEVICES WITH FDA PREMARKET APPROVAL*

Vanessa K. Burrows

SUMMARY

In *Riegel v. Medtronic, Inc.*, the United States Supreme Court held in an 8 to 1 decision that if the Food and Drug Administration (FDA) grants premarket approval (PMA) to a medical device, the device manufacturer is immune from certain suits under state tort law, due to an express preemption provision in the Medical Device Amendments of 1976 (MDA). This holding establishes that FDA PMA preempts claims such as strict liability, breach of implied warranty, and negligence in design, testing, manufacturing, labeling, distribution, sale, inspection, or marketing of the device to the extent that such state law claims are "different from, or in addition to" federal PMA requirements. However, the Supreme Court held that the MDA's express preemption provision did not prohibit state "claims premised on a violation of FDA regulation." The Court stated that such claims "'parallel,' rather than add to, federal requirements." Post-*Riegel*, the lower courts have come to differing

* This is an edited, reformatted and augmented version of Congressional Research Service, Publication No. R40534, dated January 13, 2012.

conclusions when determining whether particular state law claims, such as manufacturing defect claims, "parallel" federal requirements, and thus are not preempted, or rather are state requirements "different from, or in addition to" federal requirements, and thus are preempted under *Riegel.*

The Supreme Court's decision has been a cause for concern for some Members of Congress who disagree with the ruling, as well as trial lawyers and patients. However, advocates of more limited tort liability, including the previous Administration, agree with the ruling. The decision has broad implications for consumers of Class III medical devices, who are prevented from suing device manufacturers on most state common law claims, as well as manufacturers, who are shielded from many suits if their device receives FDA PMA. In the 111th Congress, bills were introduced—H.R. 1346, H.R. 4816, and S. 540—that would have overturned the Court's decision in *Riegel* by modifying the statute at issue. As of the date of this report, similar legislation has not been introduced in the 112th Congress.

This report will provide a brief overview of federal premarket regulation of medical devices. The report then provides an overview of federal preemption of state law, as well as arguments for and against federal preemption of state law tort claims with respect to medical devices. The report explains the Supreme Court's decision in *Riegel* and examines the concurring and dissenting opinions. Finally, the report analyzes the legal, procedural, policy, and legislative implications for Congress, consumers, and medical device manufacturers.

INTRODUCTION

In order to elucidate the Supreme Court's decision in *Riegel v. Medtronic, Inc.*,[1] this report begins by providing background on the Food and Drug Administration's (FDA's) premarket regulation of medical devices and an overview of federal preemption of state law. The report discusses arguments for and against federal preemption of state law tort claims with respect to medical devices. Next, the report examines the FDA's shifting position on federal preemption in medical device cases. The report then explains the Supreme Court's decision in *Riegel v. Medtronic, Inc.*, as well as the concurring and dissenting opinions. Finally, the report analyzes the implications of the Court's decision in *Riegel* for Congress, consumers, medical device manufacturers, and preemption jurisprudence.

This report focuses on Class III medical devices because it is federal preemption of state law requirements that are "different from, or in addition to" federal requirements for Class III devices with premarket approval (PMA) that was at issue in *Riegel.*[2]

AN OVERVIEW OF FDA PREMARKET NOTIFICATION AND PREMARKET APPROVAL (PMA) OF MEDICAL DEVICES

The Federal Food, Drug, and Cosmetic Act (FFDCA)[3] sets forth a detailed set of statutory requirements designed to ensure that medical devices are safe and effective. As a result, medical devices must meet certain minimum requirements before they may be marketed in the United States. For example, the device cannot be adulterated or misbranded, and there are registration, good manufacturing practices, and labeling requirements.[4] There are also more specific requirements that a device manufacturer must follow, which are determined by the level of risk that the device poses to patients from its use or misuse.[5]

Medical devices are classified according to risk—Class I (low risk), Class II (moderate risk), and Class III (high risk)—and there are certain requirements based on that risk.[6] Class III devices, which are those "purported or represented to be for a use in supporting or sustaining human life or for a use which is of substantial importance in preventing impairment of human health" or those that "present[] a potential unreasonable risk of illness or injury," are generally subject to premarket approval (PMA).[7] Examples of Class III devices include replacement heart valves, silicone gel-filled breast implants, and pacemaker pulse generators.[8]

All new devices are automatically designated as Class III, and therefore must receive PMA, unless the device meets one of three exceptions: (1) the "grandfather" provision for devices on the market prior to the passage of the Medical Device Amendments of 1976 (MDA),[9] (2) a device on the market after the passage of the MDA that has been classified as Class I or Class II or reclassified as Class I or Class II by the FDA after the manufacturer files a petition for reclassification,[10] or (3) the device is "substantially equivalent" to either a grandfathered device or a Class I or Class II device.[11] A device is "substantially equivalent" if the FDA makes such a determination based on a comparison of the new device with a predicate device.[12] A predicate device could have been marketed either before or after 1976.[13] The device seeking the "substantially equivalent" determination must either have (1) the same intended use[14] and the same technological characteristics as the predicate device, or (2) the same intended use, different technological characteristics, and information and data that demonstrate safety and effectiveness, and cannot "raise different questions of safety and effectiveness than the predicate device."[15] The manufacturer decides which predicate device to use for the comparison with the new device. However, the FDA has discretion in determining whether the comparison is appropriate.

Premarket Notification (§ 510(k) Submissions)

Premarket notification is known as a § 510(k) submission, after the section of the FFDCA that requires it. Class III devices generally require a premarket notification as well as PMA.

However, some Class III devices may be marketed only with a § 510(k) submission—if the device was introduced after the passage of the MDA in 1976 and is substantially equivalent to a pre-1976 device, but there is no regulation requiring PMA.[16] The majority of new Class III medical devices reach the marketplace after a § 510k submission, as opposed to the receipt of FDA PMA.[17]

Premarket notification applies to new devices that are not substantially equivalent to pre-1976 devices, devices introduced after passage of the MDA in 1976 that have been reclassified as Class I or Class II, and devices that may have been or currently are on the market, but that have been significantly modified.[18]

At least 90 days before a manufacturer may market one of these new devices, the manufacturer must submit a notification to the FDA.[19] After the FDA reviews a premarket notification under § 510(k), the agency may find that the device either is or is not substantially equivalent to a predicate device, request more information, withhold a decision pending the submission of certain information, or advise the submitter that the device does not require premarket notification.[20]

Premarket Approval (PMA)

As noted above, a PMA application is required for most Class III devices, with three exceptions.[21] In the PMA process, the FDA determines if these devices have a "reasonable assurance of ... safety and effectiveness."[22]

A PMA application must include, among other facts, information regarding proposed labeling, reports of information "concerning investigations which have been made to show whether or not such device is safe and effective," a description of the manufacturing and processing methods, samples of the device and its components, and information regarding the components, ingredients, and operating principles of the device.[23]

A PMA application will be denied approval if "there is a lack of a showing of reasonable assurance that such device is safe [and effective] under the conditions of use" in the proposed labeling; if the methods of manufacturing, processing, packing, or installing the device do not conform to good manufacturing practices; if the proposed labeling is false or misleading; or if the device does not meet performance standards.[24]

The FDA cannot disclose the existence of a PMA application file before issuing an approval order to the applicant "unless it previously has been publicly disclosed or acknowledged."[25]

PMA Supplements

Once a device has been approved through the PMA process, the manufacturer can market the device only for its intended use. For example, a device, such as a stent, approved to treat coronary artery disease may not be marketed for treatment of blocked biliary ducts unless the manufacturer files a PMA supplement for FDA review and approval.[26]

The FDA must approve the PMA supplement before the manufacturer may make a "change affecting the safety or effectiveness of the device for which the applicant has an approved PMA," such as changes to the labeling, packaging, sterilization procedures, and new indications for use of the device (as in the stent example).[27]

However, in certain cases, a change to a device with PMA "that enhances the safety of the device or the safety in the use of the device may be placed into effect by the applicant prior to the receipt ... of a written FDA order approving the PMA supplement."[28]

PREEMPTION

This section will first provide an overview of federal preemption of state law. It will then discuss arguments for and against preemption of state law tort claims with respect to medical devices. Finally, this section will discuss the change in the FDA's position on preemption in medical device cases.

Federal Preemption of State Law

The preemption doctrine is derived from the Supremacy Clause of the U.S. Constitution, which establishes that the laws of the United States "shall be the supreme law of the land; and the judges in every state shall be bound thereby, any thing in the Constitution or laws of any State to the contrary notwithstanding."[29] In applying this constitutional mandate, courts have recognized both express and implied forms of preemption, which are "compelled whether Congress' command is explicitly stated in the statute's language, or implicitly contained in its structure and purpose."[30] Both types of preemption may apply to state legislation, regulations, and common law. As the Supreme Court held in *Gade v. National Solid Wastes Management Association*, "the question whether a certain state action is pre-empted by a federal law is one of congressional intent. The purpose of Congress is the ultimate touchstone. To discern Congress' intent we examine the explicit statutory language and the structure and purpose of the statute."[31]

In the *express* preemption context, a federal statute will be deemed to supplant existing state law to the extent that it contains an explicit provision to that effect, the scope of which is determined by interpreting the language of the provision and analyzing the legislative history as necessary.[32] Where express preemption provisions are not present, federal law may preempt state law implicitly. There are several different ways to conceptualize the doctrine of *implied* preemption, but it is often subdivided into three general categories for purposes of analysis: (1) federal occupation of the entire field of regulation; (2) actual conflict between federal and state requirements; and (3) state requirements that frustrate congressional purpose.[33]

Courts, however, often encounter difficulty when federal law is silent as to the preemptive effect. The Supreme Court traditionally begins its analysis in this context with a presumption against preemption, an "assumption that the historic police powers of the States were not to be superseded by [a federal law] unless that was the clear and manifest purpose of Congress."[34] Several decisions by the Court have strengthened this presumption, including *Maryland v. Louisiana*, which stated that "[c]onsideration under the Supremacy clause starts with the basic assumption that Congress did not intend to displace state law,"[35] and *Chicago & North Western Transportation Co. v. Kalo Brick & Tile Co.*, which held that "[p]reemption of state law by federal statute or regulation is not favored 'in the absence of persuasive reasons either that the nature of the regulated subject matter permits no other conclusion, or that the Congress has unmistakably ordained.'"[36] Additionally, in the Supreme Court case *Medtronic, Inc. v. Lohr*, which also addressed preemption of state tort claims under the MDA, the plurality opinion noted:

> Throughout our history the several States have exercised their police powers to protect the health and safety of their citizens. Because these are "primarily, and historically, ... matter[s] of local concern," *Hillsborough County* v. *Automated Medical Laboratories, Inc.*, 471 U.S. 707, 719 (1985), the "States traditionally have had great latitude under their police powers to legislate as to the protection of the lives, limbs, health, comfort, and quiet of all persons." *Metropolitan Life Ins. Co.* v. *Massachusetts*, 471 U.S. 724, 756 (1985) (internal quotation marks omitted).[37]

These standards, however, are highly case specific in their application. Indeed, the Supreme Court itself has noted that "none of these expressions provide an infallible constitutional test or an exclusive constitutional yardstick. In the final analysis, there can be no crystal clear distinctly marked formula."[38] Thus, cases involving federal preemption of state law often hinge on the particular factual circumstances of a given case.

Arguments for Federal Preemption of State Law Tort Claims with Respect to Devices

There are policy arguments for and against the merits of preemption in the medical device context. Arguments for federal preemption of common law in the medical device context focus on (1) uniform national standards, (2) the rigor of the PMA process, (3) the FDA's expertise in this field, and (4) the potential for delay in the development of new products. Businesses tend to favor preemption, as regulated industries "generally prefer uniform, national regulation over varying state regulation."[39]

Those in favor of preemption, including the Pharmaceutical Research and Manufacturers of America (PhRMA) and trade groups for medical device makers such as the Advanced Medical Technology Association (AdvaMed), equate jury verdicts under state common law with the imposition of a state law "requirement" in addition to "requirements" that are imposed for devices under the FFDCA and FDA regulations.[40] For example, medical device manufacturers have argued that in light of the rigor of the FDA's PMA process[41] and its resulting "device-specific design, manufacturing, and labeling requirements," separate jury verdicts would also produce "requirements" as a practical matter with regard to a device's design, manufacture, or label.[42] One court of appeals case explained the effect of a jury verdict this way:

> The effect of a jury finding of negligent failure to warn would be that state law would require [the manufacturer] to change the label and package insert for [the medical device], but [the manufacturer] may not unilaterally make such changes under federal law. A device may not be labeled in a manner inconsistent with any conditions specified in its PMA. 21 C.F.R. § 814.80 (2000). A manufacturer must submit a Supplemental PMA for any proposed labeling changes that affect the safety of the device. *Id.* at § 814.39(a).[43]

Others in favor of preemption, such as the George W. Bush Administration, similarly have pointed to the FDA as an agency composed of expert scientists vested with authority to undertake matters such as PMA, which should not be overruled by potentially inconsistent state juries. They argue that juries lack the FDA's expertise to engage in a balancing of the benefits and risks that products may pose.[44] Finally, preemption advocates argue that to decide differently may delay or discourage development and marketing of products with beneficial or even life-saving potential, and that recalls of medical devices are "rare."[45] They also respond to the argument that preemption does not give the manufacturer the incentive to update and improve its devices by saying that market pressures will force companies to change their products.[46]

Arguments Against Federal Preemption of State Law Tort Claims with Respect to Devices

In contrast, arguments against federal preemption of common law in the medical device field focus on (1) congressional intent and legislative history, (2) protections for consumers, who may otherwise be left without a remedy, (3) the change in the FDA's view with regard to preemption, as well as the general presumption against preemption, (4) viewing FDA approval as a preliminary step—a "floor" rather than a "ceiling"—that does not hold manufacturers accountable for safety concerns, and (5) questioning the agency's capabilities in terms of resources and its reliance on industry.

With regard to congressional intent, some commentators have noted that "Congress did not directly address tort suits in the MDA, despite decades of lawsuits against drug manufacturers."[47] Opponents of federal preemption of state common law claims in the device area, such as Senator Kennedy and Congressman Waxman, have argued that Congress's silence on the issue evidences "its intent not to preempt the suits,"[48] or alternately, that the discussions in the legislative history do not provide evidence of such intent.[49] In *Riegel*, discussed below, the plaintiffs' attorney also questioned whether Congress would "have really intended to protect the manufacturer from liability," since the passage of the MDA occurred in the wake of the Dalkon Shield cases,[50] in which an intrauterine device "was linked to serious infections and several deaths, not to mention a large number of pregnancies."[51]

Some who are against preemption view tort law as an "important and necessary adjunct to the regulatory process"[52] and cite the FDA's view prior to 2004 that federal law did not preempt product liability lawsuits.[53] While proponents of preemption see it as a way to protect orderly business functions, others assert that "industry has been pushing to expand federal pre-emption for the past 25 years as a wholesale, get-out-of-jail-free card."[54] The Riegels' counsel and others have argued that FDA PMA should be seen as "a preliminary judgment of safety and effectiveness that did not relieve a manufacturer of an obligation to make a device better and safer."[55]

Moreover, as the Justices explored at oral argument in *Riegel*, preemption could shield manufacturers who discover a risk or problem with their FDA-approved device, if the FDA has not yet learned of the problem or has not taken action as a result of the risk.[56]

It could be argued that the FDA is dependent on manufacturers to provide information regarding devices, that "[t]here is no opportunity for public comment or for any public challenge to the information presented to the FDA by the device manufacturer" in the PMA application, and to allow the common law tort claims to go forward may reveal information in the discovery process that manufacturers withheld from the FDA in the PMA process.[57]

This view sees the state tort law system as a backstop, as safety concerns may "have been uncovered not by the agency but during the course of litigation."[58]

Concerns have been raised that companies may also not "respond to safety concerns that arise after a product is on the market," if federal law preempts state tort claims, or even attempt to manufacture new devices that are safer or better because suits related to marketing previously approved devices would be preempted.[59] Those who view the agency as overburdened may also similarly view the agency's PMA process as inadequate to protect patients.[60]

The FDA's Position on Preemption in Medical Device Cases

Over the years, the FDA's position on preemption of state tort law claims in medical device cases has shifted.[61] This section will discuss the express preemption provision, as well as the FDA's positions since the provision was first enacted in 1976.

The FFDCA contains an express preemption provision with respect to medical devices. This provision was included as part of the MDA, which was enacted in 1976. The statute, 21 U.S.C. § 360k(a), which was at issue in *Riegel*, provides:

> Except as provided in subsection (b) of this section, no State or political subdivision of a State may establish or continue in effect with respect to a device intended for human use any requirement—
>
> (1) which is different from or in addition to, any requirement applicable under [federal law] to the device, and
>
> (2) which relates to the safety or effectiveness of the device or to any other matter included in a requirement applicable to the device under [relevant federal law].[62]

However, the agency may exempt state requirements that are "more stringent" and state requirements "required by compelling local conditions" if "compliance with the requirement would not cause the device to be in violation of any applicable requirement under" the FFDCA.[63]

The FDA subsequently issued regulations interpreting this preemption provision in 1978, which were amended after the Supreme Court issued its decision in *Medtronic, Inc. v. Lohr.*[64] In that case, the Court concluded that state common law negligence actions against manufacturers of devices found by the FDA to be "substantially equivalent" under the § 510(k) process were not preempted. In the agency's post-*Lohr* 1996 final rule amending the regulations, the FDA noted that "the new quality system regulation does not preempt State tort and common law remedies."[65] The regulations presently provide:

> State or local requirements are preempted *only* when the Food and Drug Administration has established specific counterpart regulations or there are other specific requirements applicable to a particular device under the act, thereby making any existing divergent State or local requirements applicable to the device different from or in addition to, the specific Food and Drug Administration requirements.

> Section 521(a) [21 U.S.C. § 360k(a)] does not preempt State or local requirements of general applicability where the purpose of the requirement relates either to other products in addition to devices ... or to unfair trade practices in which the requirements are not limited to devices....[66]

As indicated by these regulations, the FDA's position, prior to the early 2000s, was of a "longstanding presumption against preemption in implementing section 521" of the FFDCA (21 U.S.C. § 360k).[67] The agency's outlook with regard to the scope of the preemption provision was that it "should be interpreted narrowly, with a presumption against preemption."[68] With regard to whether the preemption provision applied to state tort claims, the "FDA did not have occasion to address the precise issue of whether [21 U.S.C. § 360k] preempts state tort claims before that issue was litigated in private lawsuits."[69] In 1997, the then-Chief Counsel of the FDA argued that "although the agency had not formally expressed its position on the precise issue, it is clear from the views it expressed in many other contexts [such as a 1984 advisory opinion, a response to a 1980 request from California for an exemption from preemption, and a response to "a congressional request for an opinion on the preemptive status of another California statute"] that it did not believe that state tort claims were preempted under" 21 U.S.C. § 360k.[70] She referred to the statute's legislative history, the exemption procedure, and the lack of congressional mention of its intent to preempt state common law claims when noting the agency's "belie[f] that Congress intended to restrict preemption to positive enactments (for example, legislation or regulations) that apply to the marketing of medical devices within a state."[71]

Meanwhile, in *Lohr*, the agency had argued in an *amicus* brief that "state tort claims generally are not preempted under" 21 U.S.C. § 360k.[72] After the Supreme Court's decision in *Lohr*, the then-Chief Counsel for the FDA, Margaret J. Porter, stated:

> FDA regulation of a device cannot anticipate and protect against all safety risks to individual consumers. Even the most thorough regulation of a product such as a critical medical device may fail to identify potential problems presented by the product. Regulation cannot protect against all possible injuries that might result from use of a device over time. Preemption of all such claims would result in the loss of a significant layer of consumer protection, leaving consumers without a remedy for injuries caused by defective medical devices. Moreover, FDA's regulation of devices would have been accorded an entirely different weight in private tort litigation than its counterpart regulation of

> drugs and biologics. This disparity is neither justified nor appropriate, nor does the agency believe it was intended by Congress when section 521 [21 U.S.C. § 360k] was enacted.[73]

The FDA's view on preemption in medical device cases appeared to shift in 2004, when the agency filed an appellate brief in *Horn v. Thoratec Corp.*, in which the plaintiff sued the medical device manufacturer alleging negligence, defective design, defective manufacture, and failure to warn.[74] In *Horn*, the FDA submitted an *amicus curiae* letter brief to the court, which the court referenced, in which the agency "unequivocally expressed the opinion that state common law claims such as those made by Horn against a PMA-approved device are preempted."[75]

However, the shift may have occurred earlier. As the court in *Horn* noted, the FDA argued in a 2003 statement of interest in a Tennessee circuit court case that PMA "triggers preemption of a wide array of requirements imposed under state tort law."[76] Others have argued that the agency's support of preemption began even prior to the change of presidential Administrations from Bill Clinton to George W. Bush, although this assertion was not limited to medical device cases.[77] One scholar has characterized preemption "as a fundamentally political issue."[78]

In its 2004 amicus brief in *Horn*, the agency specifically acknowledged that it was disclaiming its previous view that 21 U.S.C. § 360k "does not preempt a state tort law claim concerning an FDA-approved device,"[79] which the agency had articulated in a 1997 *amicus* brief.[80] The agency gave several reasons for its change in position. The FDA previously asserted that its approval of a manufacturer's design did not "convert the features of that design into federal requirements," but now stated that such a "proposition does not adequately account for the highly detailed ... nature of the PMA process."[81] The agency also noted that its past position viewed the PMA process as a minimum standard, which "should not displace state common law that may provide additional protection to consumers," but said in its 2004 *amicus* brief that PMA "sets a ceiling as well as a floor."[82] Finally, the FDA noted that its position change "reflects in part the decisions applying *Lohr* issued by the federal courts" since the Supreme Court issued that opinion.[83]

The agency's view under the George W. Bush Administration was that state common law tort claims, such as those at issue in *Horn* and *Riegel*, are preempted under 21 U.S.C. § 360k because the FDA granted PMA, which imposes specific federal requirements on the Class III medical device at issue, and the state common law claims "would impose a requirement different from, or in addition to, the requirements imposed by FDA in granting pre-market approval."[84] The agency previously stated that even though it does not issue specific federal regulations for a device, "the agency's approval of this device through the PMA process does impose specific requirements for the product, including requirements for its design, manufacturing, performance, labeling, and use," which are based on the manufacturer's PMA application.[85] Additionally, the agency asserted that five Justices in *Lohr* "concluded that a state common law tort judgment is a 'requirement' under Section 360k(a)."[86] Therefore, under the agency's view of preemption during the Bush Administration, "any finding of liability based upon [a device manufacturer's] failure to satisfy a standard different from those approved by the FDA in the PMA process would necessarily rest upon an implicit requirement that this device be designed, manufactured, or marketed in a way that differs from the way approved by FDA."[87]

Though the *Riegel* decision was issued before the start of the Obama Administration, the President announced his policy on preemption in a 2009 memorandum, which stated that "preemption of State law by executive departments and agencies should be undertaken only with full consideration of the legitimate prerogatives of the States and with a sufficient legal basis for preemption."[88] The memorandum explicitly addressed the inclusion of preemption statements in regulatory preambles and said such statements should not be included unless the preemption provision is included in the regulation itself. Additionally, such provisions should not be included in the regulation unless they were "justified under legal principles governing preemption," including those in President Clinton's Executive Order 13132 on federalism.[89] That executive order requires agencies to "construe ... a Federal statute to preempt State law only where the statute contains an express preemption provision or there is some other clear evidence that the Congress intended preemption of State law, or where the exercise of State authority conflicts with the exercise of Federal authority under the Federal statute."[90] When addressing preemption in terms of federal requirements in recent regulations, the FDA has cited President Clinton's executive order on federalism as well as the Supreme Court's holding in *Riegel*.[91]

The Obama memorandum also called upon agencies to review regulations issued in the previous 10 years that included statements in the preamble or the regulation itself with regard to preemption of state law.[92] A 2008 *Associated Press* article noted that 51 regulations proposed or adopted since 2005 had placed limits on lawsuits and that a combined 41 of those 51 came from the FDA and the National Highway Traffic Safety Administration.[93] In 2011, the

FDA issued its preemption review. The FDA concluded that its position on preemption that had been articulated in the preamble to a rule on supplemental applications for labeling changes for prescription drugs, biologics, and devices—a position also referenced in rules on nonprescription drugs and food labeling—could not "be justified under legal principles governing preemption."[94] These legal principles included the Supreme Court's decision in *Wyeth v. Levine*, which explicitly addressed the FDA's preemption position in that labeling rule.[95]

RIEGEL V. MEDTRONIC, INC.

This section will discuss the Supreme Court's 2008 decision in *Riegel*, as well as the concurrence and the dissent. The *Riegel* case involved preemption of state common law tort suits regarding medical devices that have been FDA-approved under the PMA process.

The U.S. Supreme Court Decision

The *Riegel* case involved a catheter that had received PMA from the FDA to be marketed by Medtronic, Inc. as a Class III device.[96] The "device's labeling stated that use was contraindicated for patients with ... calcified stenoses," in other words, narrowed or constricted passages.[97]

The patient, Charles Riegel, had a "diffusely diseased and heavily calcified" right coronary artery.[98] Riegel's doctor inflated the "catheter five times, to a pressure of 10 atmospheres," although the device's labeling "warned that the catheter should not be inflated beyond its rated burst pressure of eight atmospheres."[99]

The catheter burst on the fifth inflation, and "Riegel developed a heart block, was placed on life support, and underwent emergency coronary bypass surgery. "[100] The patient and his wife raised New York state common law claims of "strict liability; breach of implied warranty; and negligence in the design, testing, inspection, distribution, labeling, marketing, and sale of the catheter."[101]

The Supreme Court found that the Medical Device Amendments of 1976 (MDA) preempted state tort law claims because the common law negligence and strict liability claims fell into the category of "any requirement" in the bolded language below. Section 360k(a) of Title 21, United States Code (FFDCA § 521) reads:

> Except as provided in subsection (b) of this section, no State or political subdivision of a State may establish or continue in effect with respect to a device intended for human use any requirement—
>
> (1) which is different from or in addition to, any requirement applicable under [federal law] to the device, and
>
> (2) which relates to the safety or effectiveness of the device or to any other matter included in a requirement applicable to the device under [relevant federal law].

In other words, the Court held that the federal government had established requirements in the PMA process for medical devices in the MDA. The Court said that the New York state common law claims were "different from or in addition to" the federal MDA requirements because "reference to a State's 'requirements' includes its common-law duties."[102]

To reach its holding, the Court addressed two questions: (1) Has the federal government established requirements applicable to the medical device? and (2) If the answer to the first question is yes, are the plaintiffs' common law claims (such as negligence in the design, labeling, and marketing of the catheter) based on state requirements that are "different from, or in addition to" the federal requirements, "and that relate to safety and effectiveness"?[103]

First, the Court held that the federal government had "established requirements applicable to" the device at issue, Medtronic's catheter, and that PMA "imposes 'requirements' under the MDA."[104] In making its determination, the Court distinguished its earlier decision in *Medtronic, Inc. v. Lohr*, which held that "federal manufacturing and labeling requirements" do not preempt common law claims of negligence and strict liability in instances where: (1) any federal requirements are not specific to the device at issue; and (2) the FDA finds that a device "is 'substantially equivalent' to another device exempt from premarket approval,"[105] because this constituted an exemption, not a "requirement."[106] The Court found that, unlike the substantial equivalence process, PMA is device-specific and is not an exemption, but rather a "requirement."[107] The Court differentiated from *Lohr* by reasoning that PMA is focused on safety, rather than equivalence; that PMA is a formal FDA review, as opposed to the lack of formal review that the device subject to premarket notification in *Lohr* received; and that devices that receive PMA may not deviate from the FDA-approved specifications in the PMA application.[108]

Second, the Court held that "New York's tort duties constitute 'requirements' under the MDA"[109] and that these "requirements" were "different from, or in addition to" the federal requirements. The Court began by noting that five Justices in *Lohr* "concluded that common-law causes of action for negligence and strict liability do impose 'requirement[s]' and would be pre-empted by federal requirements *specific* to a medical device."[110] The *Lohr* Court had said that it did "not believe that [the MDA's] statutory and regulatory language necessarily precludes ... 'general' state requirements from ever being pre-empted...."[111] In other words, the MDA could potentially preempt general state "requirements," or general state common law under circumstances such as strict liability, negligence, and implied warranty claims.[112]

The Court also addressed the Riegels' argument that general common law duties are not "requirements" specific to medical devices, and therefore should not be preempted. This argument depended on the FDA regulation 21 C.F.R. § 808.1(d)(1), which states "that MDA preemption does not extend to '[s]tate or local requirement of general applicability [whose] purpose ... relates either to other products in addition to devices.'"[113] However, the regulation also "states that the MDA sets forth a 'general rule' pre-empting state duties 'having the force and effect of law (whether established by statute, ordinance, regulation, or court decision).'"[114] It was this subsection of the regulation prompted the Court to note that only common law duties are established by court decision.[115]

Additionally, the Court undertook a discussion of the statutory text and informed Congress of the meaning that "this Court will assign to terms regularly used" in congressional enactments: "Absent other indication, reference to a State's 'requirements' includes its common-law duties."[116] The Court then remarked that "[i]n the present case, there is nothing to contradict the normal meaning" that the term "requirements" will include state common-law duties.[117] The Court then indicated that state tort law was perhaps "less deserving of preservation" than state statutes or state regulations, as one state jury could potentially "set state standards 'different from, or in addition to' federal standards."[118]

The Court held that New York's common law causes of action were preempted by the MDA "only to the extent that they are 'different from, or in addition to' the requirements imposed by federal law."[119] To the extent that the lawsuit raises claims that "'parallel' rather than add to, federal requirements," such as a state "damages remedy for claims premised on a violation of FDA regulations," it does not appear that such suits would be preempted.[120]

Justice Stevens's Concurrence

Justice Stevens agreed with the dissent's "description of the actual history and principal purpose of the pre-emption provision at issue" and observed that the text of the provision "cover[s] territory not actually envisioned by its authors."[121] He also dispensed with congressional intent in this case: "we have frequently concluded that 'it is ultimately the provisions of our laws rather than the principal concerns of our legislators by which we are governed.'"[122] However, he agreed with the majority that New York common law duties "constitute requirements with respect to the device at issue that differ from federal requirements relating to safety and effectiveness."[123] He found that the preemption provision's language "encompasses other types of 'requirements'" and that "common-law rules administered by judges ... create and define legal obligations, [therefore] some of them unquestionably qualify as 'requirements.'"[124]

Justice Ginsburg's Dissent

Justice Ginsburg's dissent focused on the intent of Congress in enacting the MDA, as well as previous Supreme Court cases emphasizing congressional intent as the "ultimate touchstone of pre-emption analysis."[125] The dissent tracks the Court's presumption against preemption analysis outlined earlier in this report and stated that "[w]here the text of a preemption clause is open to more than one plausible reading, courts ordinarily 'accept the reading that disfavors preemption.'"[126]

Beginning with the majority's holding that "[a]bsent other indication, reference to a State's 'requirements' includes its common law duties," she stated that "other indication[s]" exist in the MDA and its legislative history that preclude the Court's conclusion that the MDA preempts state common law claims.[127] Justice Ginsburg noted the act's consumer-oriented purpose, as well as congressional awareness of over 500 lawsuits related to the Dalkon Shield medical device: "I find informative the absence of any sign of a legislative design to preempt state common-law tort actions."[128] She pointed to the absence of a federal compensation scheme for consumers injured by FDA-approved medical devices as evidence that Congress did not intend to preempt state common law suits.[129] Furthermore, she referenced the Court's plurality in *Lohr*, which stated: "[N]othing in the hearings, the Committee reports, or the debates ... suggest[ed] that any proponent of the legislation intended a sweeping pre-emption of traditional common-law remedies against manufacturers and distributors of defective devices."[130] Justice Ginsburg also cited remedies provided by the MDA—such as the FDA's ability to order a device manufacturer to repair or recall the device—and a provision stating that compliance with an FDA order to recall or repair a device "shall not relieve any person from liability under Federal or State law," as evidence that Congress did not intend to preempt state common law suits.[131]

With regard to the FDA's shift in its position on preemption, she took note of the FDA's pre-2003 view, as described by a former FDA counsel, that "FDA product approval and state tort liability usually operate independently, each providing a significant, yet distinct, layer of consumer protection ... [as] [e]ven the most thorough regulation of a product ... may fail to identify potential problems."[132] The dissent then addressed the deference that should be granted to the FDA's new position on preemption, finding that the agency's announcement of its position shift in an *amicus* brief would be entitled to little deference when compared with the FDA's previous view, the presumption against preemption, and the MDA itself.[133]

The dissent next examined the history of federal regulation of medical devices, and in part, federal regulation of drugs and additives. Justice Ginsburg noted that, prior to the enactment of the MDA in 1976, the defense of state common law claims for defective design or drug labeling either did not involve preemption or, if preemption was asserted as a defense, it was unsuccessful.[134] She argues that Congress included the preemption provision 21 U.S.C. § 360k "to empower the FDA to exercise control over state premarket approval systems installed at a time when there was no preclearance at the federal level," such as the California PMA system.[135] Moreover, unlike devices, states had not developed PMA processes for drugs or additives.[136]

The dissent also quotes the FDA's former counsel as observing the disparity that would arguably arise if preemption of state common law suits existed for devices with PMA, but not drugs or biologics: "This disparity is neither justified nor appropriate, nor does the agency believe it was intended by Congress."[137] Medtronic had argued that "Congress would not have wanted state juries to second-guess the FDA's finding that a medical device is safe and effective when used as directed," however the dissent noted that the PMA process for drugs is "at least as rigorous" as that for devices, and that courts "have overwhelmingly held that FDA approval of a new drug application does not preempt state tort suits."[138] The decades in which state product liability suits for drugs and FDA approval coexisted may also be seen as an indication of congressional intent not to preempt such claims, according to the dissent.[139]

Finally, Justice Ginsburg notes that device manufacturers may have two defenses to state common law suits: implied preemption under the actual conflict theory (in other words a conflict between FDA PMA of a device and the plaintiff's case theory), and "a regulatory compliance defense based on the FDA's approval of the premarket application."[140] FDA approval could be used as "evidence that [the manufacturer] used due care in the design and labeling of the product."[141]

Legal Implications

This section addresses the types of cases that may be affected by the Court's decision in *Riegel*, identifies areas that would not be affected by this opinion, and discusses similar cases that the *Riegel* Court noted may arise in the future. The *Riegel* Court held that state common law tort claims "premised on a violation of FDA regulations," such as claims that a medical device was not manufactured according to the FDA specifications or safety processes, were not preempted by 21 U.S.C. § 360k since "the state duties in such a case 'parallel,' rather than add to, federal requirements."[142] For example, individuals would be able to bring suits alleging that a device manufacturer failed to comply with FDA requirements and that there manufacturer was negligent in designing, labeling, or manufacturing the device because the manufacturer did not follow what the FDA had approved.[143]

Riegel did not alter the Court's holding in *Lohr* that the FDA's determination that a device was substantially equivalent to one on the market did not preempt state common law claims regarding defective or negligent design or damages remedies "for violations of common-law duties when those duties parallel federal requirements."[144] The Court did not address preemption in the investigational device exemption context. Nor did the Court discuss preemption in the context of PMA supplements, which are applications "required for any change to a device subject to an approved application under [21 U.S.C. § 360e] that affects safety or effectiveness, unless such a change is a modification in a manufacturing procedure or method of manufacturing and the holder of the approved application submits a written notice" detailing the change.[145]

Justice Ginsburg noted that "[t]he Court's holding does not reach an important issue outside the bounds of this case: the preemptive effect of § 360k(a) where evidence of a medical device's defect comes to light only *after* the device receives premarket approval."[146] This issue was also mentioned by Chief Justice Roberts and Justices Kennedy, Stevens, and Souter at oral argument: "[There could be a newly discovered risk that the FDA never knew about. And, nevertheless, the claim would be preemptive."[147] Justice Ginsburg also argued that manufacturers may lack the incentive to make their devices safer once they receive PMA because they "have permission to market this product as is."[148] Medtronic's counsel responded by arguing that the FDA could withdraw approval of a device already on the market if there was a safer device in existence or allow both the newer and safer device to coexist on the market with the older device that may have more risks for some patients.[149] Congressional critics argue that the FDA's initiation of withdrawal proceedings "can be a time consuming process," as the FDA "must establish that the product no longer meets the statute's safety and efficacy requirements."[150] Relatedly, these Members note that medical device clinical trials "will not identify all of the significant risks involved in the use of the device," and that rare risks "will emerge only when a device is released into a larger and more heterogeneous population."[151]

Preemption Jurisprudence

One preemption scholar, who commented that litigants and scholars alike see preemption jurisprudence as "a muddle, a mess," saw the ruling as part of a "framework for pre-emption jurisprudence" that the Supreme Court may be attempting to create.[152] An appellate and Supreme Court practice attorney also indicated that *Riegel* and similar cases "raise recurring issues, such as whether there is a presumption against pre-emption and, if so, when it applies and how strong it is, and how much deference courts should give to the federal agency's position."[153] Although the majority opinion in *Riegel* did not address the presumption against federal preemption of state law, the Court had addressed the presumption against preemption in *Lohr*:

> Although our analysis of the scope of the pre-emption statute must begin with its text ... our interpretation of that language does not occur in a contextual vacuum. Rather that interpretation is informed by two presumptions about the nature of pre-emption.... First, because the States are independent sovereigns in our federal system, we have long presumed that Congress does not cavalierly pre-empt state-law causes of action.... Second, our analysis of the scope of the statute's pre-emption is guided by our oft-repeated comment ... that 'the purpose of Congress is the ultimate touch-stone' in every pre-emption case.[154]

Given that the *Riegel* Court did not address this traditional presumption against preemption, it could be argued that the presumption may not be as strong as previously considered.[155] However, it is important to note that the Court did not explicitly repudiate this presumption.

The Riegels had argued "that the justices have relied repeatedly on the presumption that a federal statute does not pre-empt the historic police powers of the state absent a finding of Congress' 'clear and manifest intent' to do so," and that the statutory language did not contain such intent.[156] However, "a review of the Supreme Court's various preemption holdings demonstrates that the presumption is not applied in 'all pre-emption cases,' ... and that congressional intent is certainly not the 'ultimate touchstone' in every preemption case."[157]

The FDA and Preemption Cases

This section will examine the type of deference that the agency's shifting position on preemption would likely receive if addressed by a reviewing court. The Court looked to the text of the statute when considering the FDA's own interpretation of the statute's meaning. Initially, commentators on the case predicted that the amount of deference that the Court would give to the agency's position, given the FDA's reversal in favor of preemption circa 2003-04, would be a key question, as an agency interpretation "which conflicts with the agency's earlier interpretation is 'entitled to considerably less deference than a consistently held agency view.'"[158] However, jurists may use various tools of interpretation, and the Supreme Court appeared to circumvent this question by finding clear congressional intent in favor of preemption. The Court "found it unnecessary to rely upon th[e] agency view [in support of preemption] because we think the statute itself speaks clearly to the point at issue."[159] Thus, the FDA regulation did not appear to affect how the Court chose to interpret the statute.

However, the Court noted (and the dissent agreed with the type of deference that would be given) that if it "had found the statue ambiguous, and had accorded the agency's current position deference ... *Skidmore* deference would seemingly be at issue."[160] Under *Skidmore v. Swift & Co.*, "the weight of [an administrative agency's interpretation] will depend upon the thoroughness evident in its consideration, the validity of its reasoning, its consistency with earlier and later pronouncements, and all those factors which give it power to persuade, if lacking power to control."[161] The agency's lack of consistency in this area may have been a potential cause for concern, because while the FDA under the Bush Administration supported the concept of preemption, under previous Administrations the agency had taken the opposite view.[162]

Additionally, as noted above, since the Court's decision in *Riegel* was issued, the Obama Administration has directed executive departments and agencies to avoid including statements regarding intent to preempt state law through regulations or preambles to regulations.[163] It seems likely that courts will continue to address the scope of preemption with regard to FDA statutes and regulations. In two 2011 cases, the Supreme Court addressed deference to agency interpretations generally, although preemption was not at issue in these cases.[164]

Procedural Implications

In the wake of the *Riegel* decision, cases involving medical devices that received PMA from the agency have been dismissed for failure to state a "legally cognizable claim" that would "overcome[] a preemption defense."[165] These post-*Riegel* cases appear to have been affected by two other Supreme Court cases that address pleadings standards—*Bell Atlantic Corp. v. Twombly*,[166] which was decided a few months prior to *Riegel*, and *Ashcroft v. Iqbal*,[167] which was decided after *Riegel*. These two cases have been hailed by attorneys for defendant manufacturers and bemoaned by plaintiffs' attorneys for raising the plausibility requirements for pleadings.[168] Courts have found that plaintiffs with parallel state law claims did not "plead enough facts to 'state a claim that is plausible on its face'" and survive a motion to dismiss.[169] According to one circuit judge from the United States Court of Appeals for the Eighth Circuit, "[t]he combination of the rigid application of *Twombly* and the now-articulated parallel claim exception to § 360k preemption have, in these cases, led to the dismissal of over two hundred potentially meritorious lawsuits on a technicality."[170] The significance of the pleading requirements in the context of medical device PMA preemption cases decided after *Riegel* has led one pro-plaintiff law professor to argue that Congress should amend the MDA to address "what is required for proper pleading" and *Twombly*'s "effect on plaintiff's claims."[171] Additionally, if a case survives a motion to dismiss, medical device manufacturers have argued that they should receive summary judgment from the courts under *Riegel*.[172]

In terms of the frequency of preemption post-*Riegel*, one law review article examined 75 post-*Riegel* lower court cases involving medical devices with FDA PMA.[173] The author defined rulings that "maintain[ed] a cause of action" as findings of no preemption, while preemption rulings were defined as (1) those that "dismiss[ed] all claims arising from the design, manufacture, and labeling of a medical device" and (2) dismissals of cases with claims that were "insufficiently pled" in terms of the necessary factual showings.[174] According to this study, courts found preemption in 77.3% of the cases.[175]

In terms of the types of claims that have survived post-*Riegel*, according to the article, in the 17 cases in which the courts did not find preemption, the courts considered three types of claims as "sufficiently parallel and not preempted": (1) "complaints arising from injuries suffered because of a design change without FDA approval"; (2) "claims that the manufacturer made express warranties to the consumer"; and (3) "claims of manufacturing defect."[176] While these types of claims were successful in some lower courts, they were not successful in others.[177] The author found that the first type of claim was an "infrequent factual occurrence" and that most plaintiffs would not be able to use this claim.[178] The second type of claim is based on contractual theories and may involve statements made by the manufacturer.[179] The "largest number of unpreempted parallel cases" were cases based on the third type of claim, such as those in which courts "determine[d] that the device at issue was not manufactured in conformance with the FDA's Current Good Manufacturing Practice and Quality System Regulation."[180] However, at least one federal appellate court found that such claims were preempted.[181]

The types of parallel claims that may survive in the lower courts may differ from circuit to circuit. The United States Court of Appeals for the Eighth Circuit has stated that "the contours of the parallel claim exception were not addressed in *Riegel* and are as-yet ill-defined."[182] However, there may be some commonalities, and as more courts issue decisions on parallel claims post-*Riegel*, it may be easier to predict the types of parallel claims that courts will allow. According to one law review article, in five of the federal circuit courts, "in order for a parallel cause of action to be properly alleged, the claims must be premised on a violation of federal law or deviation from federal standard. Essentially, the circuit courts conclude the common law claims must go beyond alleging violation of federal statute, and the pleadings should contain sufficient detail of how the federal regulations were violated."[183]

Regulatory Implications

The Court's decision in *Riegel* has potential implications for the agency's responsibilities, regulatory authorities, and reliance on industry-provided information. The FDA's responsibilities have increased over the years, not only in the device area, but in other regulatory areas as well, including food, drugs, and tobacco. At the same time, the agency has been identified as strapped for resources and under strain because of the large amounts of responsibility it possesses.[184] While the *Riegel* decision does not grant the FDA greater responsibilities or authorities per se, it provides the FDA with more complete control over medical devices in the sense that the FDA's approval and regulatory requirements carry greater weight than state law requirements.[185] The Court's finding that the MDA preempts state common law claims related to devices that receive FDA PMA could conceivably pressure the FDA to more stringently examine devices undergoing the PMA process.[186] However, the FDA is not required to alter its considerations of devices undergoing the PMA process due to the effect that its approval would have in terms of preempting later consumer lawsuits, such as those with regard to defectively designed devices.

The agency's reliance on industry-provided information in the medical device area has led some to argue that consumers are more vulnerable post-*Riegel*.[187] The agency may decide to address the issue of notification from manufacturers who have discovered problems with their devices after receiving PMA. One former FDA Commissioner argues that once an FDA-approved product such as a drug has a wider distribution than in controlled clinical trials, it "may have a thousand times as many users," which can lead to increased numbers of adverse events such as illness or death, necessitating new warning labels or the withdrawal of the product from the market.[188] At oral argument, Justice Kennedy discussed the possibility of a notification requirement, along the lines of an adverse event reporting requirement,[189] for device manufacturers who have discovered safer alternatives: "If the manufacturer finds just from its own laboratory experiments and not because of any data it's [sic] received from doctors and patients that there's a better way to do this, does it have the obligation to notify the FDA? Mr. Olson: I don't think so, Justice Kennedy. I think that there may be marketplace incentives."[190]

Legislative Implications

Three potential legislative implications stem from the *Riegel* case. First, some Members of Congress introduced legislation in the 111th Congress to overturn the Court's decision. Second, if Congress decided not to nullify the effect of the *Riegel* decision through legislation, one congressional approach to offer a remedy to those injured by a medical device that has received FDA PMA would be to create a victim's compensation fund. Third, future legislation that references a state's "requirements" and state common law may be affected by the Court's statements in *Riegel*.

Legislative Proposals

In the 111th Congress, bills were introduced that would have overturned the Court's decision in *Riegel* by modifying the statute at issue: H.R. 1346, H.R. 4816, and S. 540. The House Energy and Commerce Committee's Subcommittee on Health held a hearing on H.R. 1346 in the 111th Congress. Similar legislation has not been introduced in the 112th Congress.

In response to the Supreme Court's decision in *Riegel*, Representative Pallone and Senator Kennedy introduced H.R. 1346/S. 540, the Medical Device Safety Act of 2009. The bill would have effectively overturned the Court's decision in *Riegel*. The bill would have modified 21 U.S.C. § 360k by adding a provision stating that "[n]othing in this section shall be construed to modify or otherwise affect any action for damages or the liability of any person under the law of any State." The addition of that clause stated that the bill would "take effect as if included in the enactment of the [MDA]," and would "apply to any civil action pending or filed on or after the date of enactment of" the legislation, if passed. The language in H.R. 1346/S. 540 was incorporated in H.R. 4816, the Food and Drug Administration Improvement Act of 2010, in the 111th Congress, which was referred to committee but did not see further action.

The AARP, the American Association for Justice, the National Conference of State Legislatures, Public Citizen, state attorneys general, consumer groups, and several Members of Congress either supported the Riegels' case and/or support overturning the Court's decision, which some have argued impacts patients and states with strong consumer protection laws.[191] A former FDA chief counsel and the American Tort Reform Association opposed the legislation, and the latter reportedly called the bill "little more than an economic stimulus for personal injury lawyers."[192]

Creating a Victim's Compensation Fund

If Congress does not overturn the *Riegel* decision, but is interested in providing a remedy for injured medical device consumers, one approach would be to establish a compensation fund. In *Riegel*, the dissent argued that Congress would not have, "'without comment, remove[d] all means of judicial recourse' for consumers injured by FDA-approved devices."[193] The majority opinion responded by stating:

> It is not our job to speculate upon congressional motives. If we were to do so, however, the *only* indication available—the *text* of the statute—suggests that the solicitude for those injured by FDA-approved devices, which the dissent finds controlling, was overcome in Congress's estimation by solicitude for those who would suffer without new medical devices if juries were allowed to apply the tort law of 50 States to all innovations.[194] (emphasis added)

It could be argued that if Congress had intended to preempt state common law claims, it may have considered a victims' compensation fund of some sort.

In the past, Congress has created compensation schemes when it has removed an individual's ability to sue. For example, the National Vaccine Injury Compensation Program prohibits suits under state tort law against manufacturers and administrators of specified vaccines unless the claimant first files a claim for limited no-fault compensation with the National Vaccine Injury Compensation Program. Congress also created the September 11th Victim Compensation Fund of 2001, under which a victim or a victim's estate could seek no-fault compensation from the program or bring a tort action against an airline or any other party, but could not do both, except to sue "any person who is a knowing participant in any conspiracy to hijack an aircraft or commit any terrorist act."[195]

Future Legislation Referencing a State's "Requirements" and State Common Law

The *Riegel* Court held that "[a]bsent other indication, reference to a State's 'requirements' includes its common law duties."[196] It appears that the Supreme Court arrived at this conclusion based on previous Supreme Court decisions addressing the term "requirements" in the state common law context, without relying on congressional intent, the FDA's own regulation,[197] or the agency's change in its position regarding preemption, which could be a motivation for congressional legislative action. Senator Kennedy and Representative Waxman argued in their *amicus* brief that the use of the term "requirement" in one statute—the Public Health Cigarette Smoking Act of 1969, which was at issue in the 1992 Supreme Court case *Cipollone v. Liggett Group, Inc.*, and was interpreted by the Supreme Court to include common law tort claims— "does not mandate a conclusion that use of the same term in a very different statute with different goals means the same thing,"[198] as the MDA "was enacted by a different Congress at a different time."[199]

Based on this statement by the *Riegel* Court however, it appears that Congress and its legislative counsel should be aware of the use of the term "requirements" in existing statutes and proposed legislation.[200] This would appear to hold true regardless of congressional intent or when the statute was enacted, as the MDA was enacted approximately 16 years prior to the Court's analysis of the term "requirements" in *Cipollone*. It appears that Congress may have already recognized post-*Cipollone* that the use of the term "requirement" in a preemption provision could preempt product liability claims.[201] Thus, if Congress does not want to preempt state common law claims, it may be advisable to provide a specific exemption for such claims when it uses the term "requirements" in the preemption context. Congress could consider inserting savings clauses to preserve state common law claims, such as those discussed in *Geier v. American Honda Motor Co.*[202] and *Sprietsma v. Mercury Marine*.[203]

End Notes

1 552 U.S. 312 (2008).

2 21 U.S.C. § 360k(a). Preemption of tort suits related to drugs that have received FDA approval, which was at issue in *Wyeth v. Levine*, and federal preemption of state tort claims related to generic prescription drug labeling, which was at issue in *Pliva, Inc. v. Mensing*, will not be addressed in this report.

3 21 U.S.C. §§ 301 *et seq.*

4 21 U.S.C. §§ 351-52, 360; 21 C.F.R. Parts 801, 809, and 820.

5 The term "manufacturer" here includes any person, organization, or sponsor that submits a PMA application to THE FDA for a medical device.

6 21 U.S.C. § 360c.

7 21 U.S.C. § 360c(a)(1)(C)(ii).

8 21 C.F.R. § 870.3925 (replacement heart valve); 21 C.F.R. § 878.3540 (silicone gel-filled breast prosthesis); 21 C.F.R. §§ 870.3600, 870.3610 (respectively, external pacemaker pulse generator and implantable pacemaker pulse generator). *See* Riegel v. Medtronic, Inc., 552 U.S. 312, 317 (2008)(citing replacement heart valves and pacemaker pulse generators).

9 21 U.S.C. § 360c(f)(1). Approximately 1,700 different generic types of medical devices that existed on the market in 1976 were "grandfathered" in under the MDA and classified in the Code of Federal Regulations.

10 21 U.S.C. § 360c(f)(1)(A)(i)(II); 21 U.S.C. § 360c(f)(1)(B); 21 C.F.R. § 860.3(c)(3).

11 21 U.S.C. § 360c(f)(1)A)(ii).

12 21 U.S.C. § 360c(i)(1)(A).

13 21 U.S.C. § 360c(f)(1)(A).

14 Intended use and indications for use provide the basis for risk classification and, therefore, the types of studies that are required to support approval or clearance of the device, and the stringency of the regulations with which the manufacturer will have to comply.

15 21 U.S.C. § 360c(i)(1)(A).

16 *See* 21 U.S.C. §§ 360c(f)(1), 360e(b), (i).

17 Riegel v. Medtronic, Inc., 552 U.S. 312, 317 (2008).

[18] 21 C.F.R. § 807.81(a). Manufacturers may use a § 510(k) when seeking a new indication (e.g., a new population, such as pediatric use, or a new disease or condition), or when changing the design or technical characteristics.

[19] 21 U.S.C. § 360(k); FFDCA § 510(k). The submission must contain the information required in 21 C.F.R. § 807, Subpart E.

[20] 21 C.F.R. § 807.100(a).

[21] 21 U.S.C. § 360e(a). The three exceptions to the PMA requirement are: (1) devices on the market prior to the enactment of the Medical Device Amendments of 1976, 21 U.S.C. §§ 360e, 360c(f); (2) devices for which there is an investigational device exemption, 21 U.S.C § 360j(g); and (3) devices that the FDA has determined are substantially equivalent to those already on the market under the § 510(k) premarket notification process, 21 U.S.C. § 360e(b)(1)(B).

[22] 21 U.S.C. § 360c(a)(C).

[23] 21 U.S.C. § 360e(c)(1). In contrast to a § 510(k) submission, PMAs generally require some clinical data.

[24] 21 U.S.C. § 360e(d)(2); 21 C.F.R. Part 814.

[25] 21 C.F.R. § 814.9(b); *see also* 21 C.F.R. §§ 814.9(e)-(f). "Upon issuance of an order approving, or an order denying approval of any PMA, FDA will make available to the public the fact of the existence of the PMA." 21 C.F.R. § 814.9(e).

[26] 21 C.F.R. § 814.39(a).

[27] 21 C.F.R. § 814.39(a); 21 U.S.C. § 360e(d)(6).

[28] 21 C.F.R. § 814.39(d)(1).

[29] U.S. CONST. art. VI, cl. 2.

[30] Gade v. National Solid Wastes Management Association, 505 U.S. 88, 97 (1992) (quoting Jones v. Rath Packing Co., 430 U.S. 519, 525 (1977)).

[31] *Id.* at 96 (internal quotation marks and case citations omitted).

[32] *Jones*, 430 U.S. at 525.

[33] Sprietsma v. Mercury Marine, 537 U.S. 51, 64 (2002); *see also* Hines v. Davidowitz, 312 U.S. 52, 61, 77 (1941) (regarding field and frustration of purpose preemption); Florida Lime and Avocado Growers, Inc. v. Paul, 373 U.S. 132, 142-43 (1963) (regarding conflict preemption).

[34] *See* Wisconsin Public Intervenor v. Mortier, 501 U.S. 597, 605 (1991); *see also* Rice v. Santa Fe Elevator Corp., 331 U.S. 218, 230 (1947).

[35] 451 U.S. 725, 746 (1981).

[36] 450 U.S. 311, 317 (1981) (quoting Florida Lime & Avocado Growers, Inc. v. Paul, 373 U.S. 132, 142 (1963)).

[37] 518 U.S. 470, 475 (1996).

[38] *Hines,* 312 U.S. at 67.

[39] Marcia Coyle, *High Stakes for Regulated Industry in Supreme Court Pre-emption Cases*, The National Law Journal, Nov. 30, 2007. One court stated that "[t]he legislative history indicates that [national uniformity] was the reason the preemption provision was included within the MDA. H.R. Rep. No. 853, 45 (1976) ("If a substantial number of differing requirements applicable to a medical device are imposed by jurisdictions other than the Federal government, interstate commerce would be unduly burdened.")." Brooks v. Howmedica, 273 F.3d 785, 797 (8th Cir. 2001).

[40] *See* Samuel Loewenberg, *Lawmakers Try to Remove Tort Shield*, Politico, June 18, 2008; Press Release, PhRMA, PhRMA Statement on Federal Preemption (June 11, 2008), http://www.phrma.org/news_room/press_releases/

phrma_statement_on_federal_preemption. The U.S. Chamber of Commerce argued that the MDA's "express preemption provision is deliberately broad." Coyle, *supra* note 39.

[41] "The FDA scrutiny process takes years and millions of dollars to prove a device's safety and efficacy. ... companies emerge only to be sued when something goes wrong, as is prone to happen in patients with serious medical conditions and with devices more technologically advanced than ever." Editorial, *Medical Double Jeopardy*, Wall Street Journal, Mar. 1, 2008, at A8.

[42] Coyle, *supra* note 39 (discussing the arguments of Medtronic's attorneys in *Riegel*).

[43] Brooks v. Howmedica, 273 F.3d 785, 796 (8th Cir. 2001).

[44] Shannon P. Duffy, *Pre-emption Issue Weighed in Label Cases*, The Legal Intelligencer, Dec. 14, 2007; Linda Greenhouse, *Supreme Court Hears Medical Device Case*, N.Y. Times, Dec. 5, 2007; Anna Edney, *High Court Case Will Define Parameters of 1976 Medical Law*, Congress Daily AM; Sam Baker, *Supreme Court Hears Arguments in FDA Preemption Case; Breyer Seen as Swing Vote*, FDA Week. At oral argument in *Riegel*, Justice Kennedy "noted that the FDA is 'specifically charged with weighing the risks against the probable benefits,' and in a state product liability case, 'the jury is doing the same thing that the FDA did.'" Laurel Newby, *Supreme Court Argument Report: Justices Mull Pre-emption of Product Liability Claims*, Law.com, Dec. 5, 2007.

[45] Greenhouse, *supra* note 44; Edney, *supra* note 44; Newby, *supra* note 44; Riegel v. Medtronic, Inc., 552 U.S. 312 (2008), Amicus Brief for AdvaMed and DRI, 2007 U.S. S. Ct. Briefs LEXIS 1290, at *1.

[46] Baker, *supra* note 44.

[47] Baker, *supra* note 44.

[48] *Id.*

[49] Brief for Amici Curiae Senator Kennedy and Congressman Waxman, Riegel v. Medtronic, Inc., 552 U.S. 312 (2008); 2007 U.S. S. Ct. Briefs LEXIS 644, at *3.

[50] Newby, *supra* note 44.

[51] Riegel v. Medtronic, 552 U.S. 312, 315 (2008).

[52] Duffy, *supra* note 44.

[53] Greenhouse, *supra* note 44. Deputy solicitor general Edwin S. Kneedler argued that the FDA's policy change on preemption "recognized that there would be a serious undermining of F.D.A.'s approval authority and its balancing of the risks and benefits if a state jury could reweigh those." *Id.* At oral argument in *Riegel*, the government asserted that it "filed a brief in - - late 1997 taking a position that PMA approval did *not* ... have preemptive effect." (emphasis added). Transcript of Oral Argument at 45, Riegel v. Medtronic, Inc., 552 U.S. 312 (2008), http://www.supremecourtus.gov/ oral_arguments/argument_transcripts/06-179.pdf. According to the government, at approximately the same time the agency issued a proposed rule—that it withdrew seven months later—and that proposed rule asserted that PMA approval did *not* have preemptive effect. *Id.*

[54] Coyle, *supra* note 39.

[55] Greenhouse, *supra* note 44; Baker, *supra* note 44.

[56] Greenhouse, *supra* note 44; *see infra* notes 146-48.

[57] Kennedy v. Collagen Corp., 67 F.3d 1453, 1456 (9th Cir. 1995); Baker, *supra* note 44; *see also* Editorial, *Our View on Pharmaceutical Safety: If a drug has FDA's OK, should you be able to sue?*, USA Today, Apr. 25, 2008 (noting that Merck, which made Vioxx, "apparently downplayed evidence that the medicine tripled the death risk in Alzheimer'sprone patients").

[58] Lawrence O. Gostin, *Reply*, J. AM. MED. ASS'N 1882 (Oct 23, 2008).

[59] Baker, *supra* note 44; *see infra* notes 146-48.

[60] *See* Gardiner Harris, *Justices Add Legal Complications to Debate on F.D.A.'s Competence*, N.Y. Times, Feb. 21, 2008, at C4; Karl Thiel, *Supreme Court Actions Add Pressure to Beleaguered FDA*, Bioworld Today, Vol. 19, Issue 42, Mar. 3, 2008. Congress has held multiple hearings on the FDA's lack of resources as compared to its obligations. *See, e.g.*, *Should FDA Drug and Medical Device Regulation Bar State Liability Claims?: Hearing Before the H. Comm. on Oversight and Gov't Reform*, 110th Cong., May 14, 2008.

[61] Former FDA Commissioner Donald Kennedy has argued that the "notion of preemption has taken on an entirely new guise, also involving the FDA, but in a far more troubling way than the older use of preemption in the regulatory sense." Donald Kennedy, Editorial, *Misbegotten Preemptions*, 320 SCIENCE 585 (May 2, 2008). He asserts that the FDA used preemption in the late 1970s, when he was commissioner of the agency, in a way that prevented states from establishing their own requirements, such as "net weight requirements for packaged foods" that may "disfavor our-ofstate competition," or their "own drug approval agenc[ies]." *Id.*

[62] 21 U.S.C. § 360k(a); FFDCA § 521(a).

[63] 21 U.S.C. § 360k(b).

[64] 43 Fed Reg. 18665 (May 2, 1978); 45 Fed. Reg. 67336 (Oct. 10, 1980); 61 Fed. Reg. 52606, 52654 (Oct. 7, 1996).

[65] 61 Fed. Reg. 52601, 52603 (Oct. 7, 1996).

[66] 21 C.F.R. § 808.1(d) (emphasis added).

[67] Margaret J. Porter, *The* Lohr *Decision: FDA Perspective and Position*, 52 FOOD & DRUG L.J. 7, 7 (1997).

[68] *Id.*

[69] *Id.* at 8.

[70] *Id.*

[71] *Id.* at 8-9.

[72] *Id.* at 10.

[73] Brief for Amici Curiae Senator Kennedy and Congressman Waxman, Riegel v. Medtronic, 552 U.S. 312 (2008); 2007 U.S. S. Ct. Briefs LEXIS 644, at *20-*21 (quoting Porter, *supra* note 67, at 11). Justice Ginsburg also quoted portions of the above paragraph in her dissent in *Riegel*, noting that "the FDA's long-held view on the limited preemptive effect of § 360k(a) better comports with the presumption against preemption of state health and safety protections, as well as the purpose and history of the MDA." Riegel v. Medtronic, Inc., 552 U.S. 312, 338 n.8 (2008) (Ginsburg, J. dissenting).

[74] 376 F.3d 163, 165 (3d Cir. 2004).

[75] *Id.* at 171.

[76] *Id.* at 171 n. 13; *see also id.* at 178.

[77] Drug and Device Law, The FDA's Amicus Curiae Briefs on Preemption—Redux, http://druganddevicelaw.blogspot.com/2007_10_01_archive.html.

[78] Samuel Raymond, *Judicial Politics and Medical Device Preemption After* Riegel, 5 NYU J. L. & LIBERTY 745, 752 (2010). *See generally* Jennie Holman Blake, *Presidential Power Grab or Pure State Might? A Modern Debate Over Executive Interpretations on Federalism*, 2000 B.Y.U.L. Rev. 293 (discussing executive orders issued by Presidents Reagan and Clinton on federal preemption of state law).

[79] Brief for Amicus Curiae U.S. Dep't of Justice, Horn v. Thoratec Corp., 376 F.3d 163 (3d Cir. 2000) (No. 02-4597), at 3, 28.

[80] Smiths Industries Medical Systems, Inc. v. Kernats, *cert. denied*, 522 U.S. 1044 (1998).

[81] Brief for Amicus Curiae U.S. Dep't of Justice, Horn v. Thoratec Corp., 376 F.3d 163 (3d Cir. 2000) (No. 02-4597), at 28.
[82] *Id.* at 29.
[83] *Id.* at 30.
[84] Brief for Amicus Curiae U.S. Dep't of Justice, Horn v. Thoratec Corp., 376 F.3d 163 (3d Cir. 2000) (No. 02-4597), at 1-2, 15.
[85] *Id.* at 15-16.
[86] *Id.* at 19.
[87] *Id.* at 18.
[88] President Obama, Memorandum for the Heads of Executive Departments and Agencies, Preemption (May 20, 2009).
[89] *Id.*
[90] Exec. Order No. 13132, 64 Fed. Reg. 43255 (Aug. 10, 1999).
[91] *See, e.g.*, FDA, Medical Devices; Ovarian Adnexal Mass Assessment Score Test System; Labeling; Black Box Restrictions, 76 Fed. Reg. 82129, 82131 (Dec. 30, 2011).
[92] President Obama, Memorandum for the Heads of Executive Departments and Agencies, Preemption (May 20, 2009).
[93] Pete Yost, *Bush Administration Uses Bureaucracy to Limit Lawsuits*, Law.com, May 14, 2008, http://www.law.com/ jsp/law/LawArticleFriendly.jsp?id=1202421377252. An FDA spokesperson stated that "[t]he preambles to these rules do not seek to preempt, but instead describe the scope of preemption under operation of federal law. *Id.* According to the article, "[j]udges have cited the FDA's regulatory preamble in its prescription drug rule in more than a dozen favorable rulings for pharmaceutical companies," although "judges have ruled for the consumers' right to sue about as often as they have ruled against them in cases touching on the regulatory preamble for prescription drug labels." *Id.*
[94] FDA, Preemption Review, 76 Fed. Reg. 61565 (Oct. 5, 2011).
[95] *Id.* at 61565.
[96] Riegel v. Medtronic, Inc., 552 U.S. 312, 310 (2008).
[97] *Id.*
[98] *Id.*
[99] *Id.*
[100] 552 U.S. at 320.
[101] *Id.*
[102] *Id.* at 324, 335.
[103] *Id.* at 321-22.
[104] *Id.* at 322-23.
[105] *Id.* at 317, 322.
[106] *Id.* at 322.
[107] *Id.* at 322-23.
[108] *Id.*
[109] *Id.* at 323.
[110] *Id.* at 323-24 (emphasis added).
[111] *Id.* at 328 n.6 (quoting Medtronic, Inc. v. Lohr, 518 U.S. 470, 500 (1996)).
[112] *Id.* at 327. The *Riegel* Court also referred to two other cases—*Bates v. Dow Agrosciences LLC*, 544 U.S. 431 (2005), and *Cipollone v. Liggett Group, Inc.*, 505 U.S. 504 (1992)—in which the Court held that statutory language regarding preemption of state "requirements" was the equivalent of preemption of state common law. *Riegel*, 552 U.S. 312, 324. In *Bates*, the Court stated: "A requirement is a rule of law that must be obeyed; an event, such as a

jury verdict, that merely motivates an optional decision is not a requirement." 544 U.S. at 445. In *Cipollone*, the Court held that a preemption provision, which prohibited states from imposing any requirement or prohibition based on smoking and health with respect to the advertising or promotion of cigarettes that are labeling in conformity with the Federal Cigarette Labeling and Advertising Act, was intended to preempt some common law claims.

[113] 21 C.F.R. § 808.1(d)(1).

[114] 21 C.F.R. § 808.1(b).

[115] *Riegel*, 552 U.S. at 329.

[116] *Id.* at 324.

[117] *Id.*

[118] *Id.* at 325.

[119] *Id.* at 330.

[120] *Id.* The Court declined to address whether the Riegels raised parallel claims, as the Riegels did not make that argument in their briefs to the Second Circuit or in their petition for certiorari. *Id.*

[121] Riegel v. Medtronic, Inc., 552 U.S. 312, 331 (Stevens, J. concurring). Justice Stevens also noted that the majority opinion advanced several policy arguments regarding impediments to development of devices.

[122] *Id.* (quoting Oncale v. Sundowner Offshore Services, Inc., 523 U.S. 75, 79-80 (1998)).

[123] *Riegel*, 552 U.S. at 332 (Stevens, J. concurring).

[124] *Id.*

[125] *Riegel*, 552 U.S. at 334 (Ginsburg, J. dissenting) (quoting Cipollone v. Liggett Group, Inc., 505 U.S. 504, 516 (1992)).

[126] *Id.* at 335 (quoting Bates v. Dow Agrosciences LLC, 544 U.S. 431, 449 (2005)).

[127] *Id.* at 335.

[128] *Id.* at 336-37.

[129] *Id.* at 337.

[130] *Riegel*, 552 U.S. at 337 n.7 (Ginsburg, J. dissenting) (quoting Medtronic, Inc. v. Lohr, 518 U.S. 470, 491 (1996)).

[131] *Id.* at 339.

[132] *Id.* at 337-38 (quoting Porter, *supra* note 67, at 11).

[133] *Id.* at 338 n.8 (examining the deference that should be accorded to the FDA's position in light of the seminal Supreme Court administrative law cases *Skidmore v. Swift & Co.* and *United States v. Mead Corp.*).

[134] *Id.* at 340 n.11.

[135] *Id.* at 341-42.

[136] *Id.* at 342.

[137] *Id.* at 340 n.12 (quoting Porter, *supra* note 67, at 11). The FFDCA is a statute with many similarities in how it regulates food, drugs, and devices. For example, the act's enforcement provisions are based on findings that a food, drug, or device is adulterated or misbranded. If a product is adulterated or misbranded, criminal and civil penalties may apply, and the agency may seek injunctions, seizures, and debarment.

[138] *Id.* at 343-44.

[139] *Id.*

[140] *Id.* at 344-45.

[141] *Id.* at 345.

[142] *Riegel*, 552 U.S. at 330; Linda Greenhouse, *Justices Shield Medical Devices from Lawsuits*, N.Y. Times, Feb. 21, 2008, at A1.

[143] Transcript of Oral Argument at 33-34, Riegel v. Medtronic, Inc., 552 U.S. 312 (2008), http://www.supremecourtus.gov/oral_arguments/argument_transcripts

[144] Medtronic, Inc. v. Lohr, 518 U.S. 470, 495 (1996).

[145] 21 U.S.C. § 360e(d)(6)(A)(i). Devices with PMA supplements include devices such as Medtronic's Sprint Fidelis pacemaker lead, which was recalled by the company since it was "more prone to developing potentially deadly fractures than an older lead called the Quattro." Barnaby J. Feder, *Medical Device Ruling Redraws Lines on Lawsuits*, N.Y. Times, Feb. 22, 2008, at C2.

[146] *Riegel*, 552 U.S. at 333 n.1 (Ginsburg, J. dissenting).

[147] Transcript of Oral Argument at 28 (Stevens, J. speaking), Riegel v. Medtronic, Inc., 552 U.S. 312 (2008), http://www.supremecourtus.gov/oral_arguments/argument_transcripts *see also id.* at 29 (Souter, J. speaking); *id.* at 26-27 (Chief Justice Roberts: "What if the FDA hasn't done it [weighed safety and effectiveness of a device versus availability]? How are newly discovered flaws dealt with? I mean, say where you have this catheter, and the FDA didn't look at the possibility of allergic reactions to the balloon plastic, and all of a sudden it turns out to be a serious problem. How can you say that that's preemptive?" Mr. Olson [Counsel for Medtronic, Inc.]: "This is a continuous process. Information must be given by the manufacturer. There is a process by which doctors report consequences to the FDA. Citizens may report information." Justice Kennedy: "Is the manufacturer free to continue to sell the device after newly discovered risks ... pending the FDA's acting on the same information?" Mr. Olson: "Yes, Justice Kennedy.")

[148] *Id.* at 35-36.

[149] *Id.* at 36.

[150] Brief for Amici Curiae Senator Kennedy and Congressman Waxman, Riegel v. Medtronic, Inc., 552 U.S. 312 (2008); 2007 U.S. S. Ct. Briefs LEXIS 644, at *19-*20.

[151] *Id.* at *19.

[152] Coyle, *supra* note 39.

[153] *Id.*

[154] Medtronic, Inc. v. Lohr, 518 U.S. 470, 485-86 (1996).

[155] While Justice Ginsburg's dissent does not criticize the Court for omitting a discussion of this presumption, she outlines the Court's typical method of analyzing cases with this presumption. Riegel v. Medtronic, Inc., 552 U.S. 312, 334-35 (2008) (Ginsburg, J. dissenting).

[156] Coyle, *supra* note 39.

[157] *See* Jodie M. Gross and Judi Abbott Curry, *The Federal Preemption Debate in Pharmaceutical Labeling Product Liability Actions*, 43 TORT TRIAL & INSURANCE PRACTICE L. J. 35, 42 (Fall 2007), (quoting Retail Clerks Int'l Ass'n Local 1625 v. Schermerhorn, 375 U.S. 96, 103 (1963) ("[T]he purpose of Congress is the ultimate touchstone.")); Raymond, *supra* note 78, at 749 (arguing that "the Court has inconsistently approved the use of a background canon of interpretation providing for a 'presumption against preemption'" and stating that while the Court did not address the presumption in *Riegel*, it "relied heavily upon it" in a subsequent Supreme Court case involving preemption of tort suits related to drugs that have received FDA approval, "to deny preemption.").

[158] Immigration & Naturalization Serv. v. Cardoza-Fonseca, 480 U.S. 421, 447 n.30 (1987); *see, e.g.*, Greenhouse, *supra* note 44. With regard to the FDA's views on preemption in drug labeling products liability cases, see Gross and Curry, *supra* note 157, at 39, which

discusses the conclusions of several courts "that FDA interpretations of its own statutes, as expressed in numerous amicus briefs as well as the preamble [to the regulation in which the FDA stated its belief that FDA approval of drug labeling preempts state law that conflicts or contradicts approved labeling], do not warrant *Chevron* deference."

[159] *Riegel*, 552 U.S. at 326.

[160] *Id.* at 326.

[161] 323 U.S. 134, 140 (1944).

[162] *See, e.g.*, *Riegel*, 552 U.S. at 326-27.

[163] President Obama, Memorandum for the Heads of Executive Departments and Agencies, Preemption (May 20, 2009).

[164] In *Pliva, Inc. v. Mensing*, the Court deferred to THE FDA's interpretation of its regulations on drug labeling. 564 U.S. __ (2011), 131 S. Ct. 2567 (2011). In *Talk America, Inc. v. Michigan Bell Telephone Co.*, the Court stated, "we defer to an agency's interpretation of its regulations, even in a legal brief, unless the interpretation is 'plainly erroneous or inconsistent with the regulation[s]' or there is any other 'reason to suspect that the interpretation does not reflect the agency's fair and considered judgment on the matter in question.'" 564 U.S. __ (2011), 131 S. Ct. 2254 (2011)(quoting Auer v. Robbins, 519 U.S. 452, 461, 462 (1997)).

[165] *See, e.g.*, Funk v. Stryker Corp., 631 F.3d 777, 779, 783 (5th Cir. 2011); Raymond, *supra* note 78, at 766-72.

[166] 550 U.S. 544 (2007).

[167] 556 U.S. 662 (2009).

[168] *See, e.g.*, Drug and Device Law Blog, http://druganddevicelaw.blogspot.com/search?q=TwIqbal+; Demetria D. Frank-Jackson, *The Medical Device Federal Preemption Trilogy: Salvaging Due Process for Injured Patients*, 35 S. ILL. U. L. J. 453 (2011).

[169] *Stryker Corp.*, 631 F.3d at 782 (quoting Ashcroft v. Iqbal); *see* Frank-Jackson, *supra* note 168, at 477-79 (stating that "claims are dismissed because the pleaders lack details in their allegations about what specific federal law the medical device manufacturer violated," and that "courts readily dismiss claims where the plaintiff's complaint fails to [establish a causal] link [between] the federal violation [and] the injury sustained by the device recipient").

[170] In re: Medtronic, Inc., Sprint Fidelis Leads Prods. Liab. Litig., 23 F.3d 1200, 1210 (8th Cir. 2010)(Melloy, J. concurring in part and dissenting in part). The judge argued that "[i]f plaintiffs must allege that the defendant violated a particular FDA-approved specification before discovery, then it is difficult to appreciate how any plaintiff will ever be able to defeat a Rule 12(b)(6) motion [to dismiss]. In essence, application of *Twombly* in this manner eliminates the remaining exception to § 360(k) preemption." *Id.* at 1212.

[171] Frank-Jackson, *supra* note 168, at 495.

[172] *See, e.g.*, Dorsey v. Allergan, Inc. and Allergan Sales, LLC, 2009 U.S. Dist. LEXIS 26235 (D. Tenn. Mar. 11, 2009) (awarding summary judgment to the breast implant manufacturer on a strict liability claim because the silicone implants, a Class III device, later received FDA PMA, even though they had not received PMA at the time of the patient's surgery). *But see* Kavalir v. Medtronic, Inc., 2008 U.S. Dist. LEXIS 82979 (N.D. Ill. Aug. 27, 2008) (denying the medical device manufacturer's motion to dismiss the patient's claims of strict liability, breach of warranty, and breach of implied warranty with regard to an implantable cardioverter defibrillator device (ICD), a Class III device, because there was not a sufficient basis to determine whether the forms of the ICDs that received PMA were the same as the

ones implanted in the plaintiff or whether the plaintiff's state tort claims were different from or in addition to FDA requirements).

[173] Raymond, *supra* note 78, at 757 (analyzing lower court cases from the date of the *Riegel* decision on February 20, 2008 through July 15, 2010).

[174] *Id.* at 758, 770-71.

[175] *Id.* at 760. The article also found that one state court "rejected" the *Riegel* decision in an opinion "explicitly calling for" congressional action. *Id.* at 756.

[176] *Id.* at 748, 766.

[177] *Id.* at 766.

[178] Raymond, *supra* note 78, at 766-67.

[179] *Id.* at 767-68.

[180] *Id.* at 768-69.

[181] *Id.* at 769-70; In re: Medtronic, Inc., Sprint Fidelis Leads Prods. Liab. Litig., 623 F.3d 1200 (8th Cir. 2010). Interestingly, the Eighth Circuit's decision was issued after Medtronic settled "all pending U.S. claims alleging product liability defects in its Sprint Fidelis defibrillator leads" in pacemakers. Alison Frankel, *8th Circuit Affirms Pre-emption Dismissal of Defibrillator Cases Against Medtronic*, American Lawyer, Oct. 21, 2010.

[182] *Sprint Fidelis*, 623 F.2d at 1204.

[183] Frank-Jackson, *supra* note 168, at 472.

[184] "The Institute of Medicine, the Government Accountability Office and the FDA's own science board have all issued reports concluding that poor management and scientific inadequacies have made the agency incapable of protecting the country against unsafe drugs, medical devices and food." Harris, *supra* note 60. The agency has countered that it is "responding to reports of its deficiencies and improving." *Id.*

[185] Supporters of the ruling, such as the Advanced Medical Technology Association, emphasize the FDA's "ultimate regulatory authority" with regard to medical devices, as opposed to multiple state regulation schemes and jury verdicts. Stephen Langel, *Democrats Threaten Legislation to Overturn Medical Device Ruling*, Congress Now, Feb. 21, 2008.

[186] Supporters have argued that the decision prevents "unscientific state juries second-guessing F.D.A.'s science-based decisions." Harris, *supra* note 60.

[187] Harris, *supra* note 60.

[188] Donald Kennedy, *Misbegotten Preemptions*, 320 SCIENCE 585 (May 2, 2008).

[189] *See, e.g.*, 21 C.F.R. Part 803, Medical Device Reporting (For example, 21 C.F.R. § 803.50(a) requires manufacturers to report to the FDA, within 30 calendar days, information that the manufacturer "receive[s] or otherwise become[s] aware of ... from any source, that reasonably suggests that a device that [the manufacturer] market[s]: (1) May have caused or contributed to a death or serious injury; or (2) Has malfunctioned and this device or a similar device that [the manufacturer] market[s] would be likely to cause or contribute to a death or serious injury, if the malfunction were to recur.").

[190] Transcript of Oral Argument at 36, Riegel v. Medtronic, Inc., 552 U.S. 312 (2008), http://www.supremecourtus.gov/ oral_arguments/argument_transcripts/06-179.pdf. Chief Justice Roberts noted that manufacturers must "disclose unpublished reports of data from clinical investigations or nonclinical laboratory studies involving the device"; however, this appears to differ from Justice Kennedy's observation regarding the obligation of a device manufacturer that has discovered or created a safer device than the one already on the market. *Id.* at 35-37.

[191] Coyle, *supra* note 39; Anna Edney, *High Court Ruling Spurs New Debate on FDA Approvals*, Congress Daily PM, Feb. 22, 2008; Inside Washington Publishers, *Michigan Governor*

Calls for Reversal of Tough Preemption Law, FDA Week, Feb. 1, 2008; Press Release, Public Citizen, Congress Must Pass Medical Device Safety Act, Restore Patient Access to Courts (Mar. 5, 2009), http://www.citizen.org/hot_issues Bill Swindell, *Trial Lawyers Lay Out Agenda for '09, Press Pre-Emption*, Congress Daily PM, Jan. 12, 2009.

[192] Marisa McQuilken, *House Hears Testimony on Medical Device Bill that Would Reverse Supreme Court Ruling*, National Law Journal, May 14, 2009.

[193] Riegel v. Medtronic, Inc., 552 U.S. 312, 337 (2008) (Ginsburg, J. dissenting).

[194] *Id.* at 326. Justice Scalia did note that "[c]ontrary to Justice Stevens' contention ... we do not 'advance' this argument [that the text of the statute is the only indication of congressional intent]. We merely suggest that if one were to speculate upon congressional purposes, the best evidence for that would be found in the statute." *Id.* at 326, n. 5.

[195] *See* CRS Report 95-797, *Federal Tort Reform Legislation: Constitutionality and Summaries of Selected Statutes*, by Vivian S. Chu; *see also* CRS Report RL33927, *Selected Federal Compensation Programs for Physical Injury or Death*, coordinated by Sarah A. Lister and C. Stephen Redhead (describing federal programs that "compensate or assist individuals who have suffered physical or psychological harm as a consequence of specific events (including the actions of others), or who have suffered specific types of physical or psychological harm").

[196] *Riegel*, 552 U.S. at 324.

[197] *Id.* at 327-29. "Even assuming that this regulation could play a role in defining the MDA's preemptive scope, it does not provide unambiguous support for the Riegels' position." *Id.* at 328. "All in all, we think that § 808.1(d)(1) can add nothing to our analysis but confusion. Neither accepting nor rejecting the proposition that this regulation can properly be consulted to determine the statute's meaning; and neither accepting nor rejecting the FDA's distinction between general requirements that directly regulate and those that regulate only incidentally; the regulation fails to alter our interpretation of the text insofar as the outcome of this case is concerned." *Id.* at 329. In contrast, the *Riegel* Court recognized that "[i]n *Lohr*, a majority of this Court interpreted the MDA's pre-emption provision in a manner 'substantially informed' by the FDA regulation set forth at 21 CFR § 808.1(d)." *Id.* at 322.

[198] Brief for Amici Curiae Senator Kennedy and Congressman Waxman, Riegel v. Medtronic, Inc., 552 U.S. 312 (2008); 2007 U.S. S. Ct. Briefs LEXIS 644, at *7-*8.

[199] *Id.* at *15.

[200] *See* Linda Greenhouse, *Supreme Court Hears Medical Device Case*, N.Y. Times, Dec. 5, 2007, at C3.

[201] Brief for Amici Curiae Senator Kennedy and Congressman Waxman, Riegel v. Medtronic, Inc., 552 U.S. 312 (2008); 2007 U.S. S. Ct. Briefs LEXIS 644, at *17 (noting that post-*Cipollone*, "Congress began explicitly stating in statutes that the term 'requirement' in preemption provisions did not preempt product liability actions. In two amendments to the FFDCA since 1992, in which Congress preempted state 'requirements,' Congress explicitly stated that product liability cases were not preempted.").

[202] 529 U.S. 861 (2000). In *Geier*, the Supreme Court held that a federal motor vehicle safety standard preempted a state common law action against a manufacturer for negligence for failure to equip a vehicle with a driver's side airbag. According to the Court, the express preemption provision of the National Traffic and Motor Vehicle Safety Act, which prohibits states from applying "any safety standard" different from an applicable federal standard, did not by itself preempt the state tort action. *Id.* at 865, 867. Preemption by statute was inconsistent with the statute's "saving clause," which provides that "compliance with" a federal safety standard "does not exempt any person from any liability under common law."

Id. at 868. This saving clause, however, did not foreclose or limit the operation of ordinary preemption principles governing override of state laws—including common law tort rules—that conflict with federal statutes or regulations. Rather, the Court held, application of the tort rule would actually conflict with the vehicle safety standard because it would operate to frustrate the objectives of the federal regulation.

[203] Unlike the decision in *Geier*, however, the Court's pronouncement on federal preemption of a state tort law claim in *Sprietsma v. Mercury Marine* upheld the common law action in the face of a preemption challenge. 537 U.S. 51 (2002). In *Sprietsma*, the Court held that the Federal Boat Safety Act of 1971 does not preempt a state common law tort action for damages from the manufacturer of an outboard motor not equipped with a propeller guard. The statute contained an express preemption clause prohibiting states from adopting or enforcing "a law or regulation ... not identical to a regulation prescribed under [the Act]." *Id.* at 59. No federal regulation requires propeller guards on outboard motors; the Coast Guard studied the matter and decided not to issue a regulation. Using basic principles of statutory construction, the Court concluded that the statute's preemption language did not encompass common law claims. The Court found that the statute's saving clause, providing that compliance with the federal standards or regulations "does not relieve a person from liability at common law," supported this conclusion. *Id.*

Index

D

E

F

G

H

I

N

O

P

Q

R

S

T

U

V

W